The AI Cure

How Artificial Intelligence is Revolutionizing Medicine

By
Dr. Julian Hawke

The AI Cure

How Artificial Intelligence is Revolutionizing Medicine

Table of Contents

Introduction

As we embark on a journey at the confluence of innovation and healthcare, it's evident that artificial intelligence (AI) is quickly transforming the landscape of medicine. Not too long ago, ideas about AI-driven healthcare belonged more to the realm of science fiction than reality. Yet today, AI is not only feasible but also significantly impactful across various facets of healthcare. This transformation is not just about futuristic visions; it's about tangible change happening as we speak, reshaping clinical practices, altering patient experiences, and redefining healthcare outcomes.

Advancements in AI are moving at a rapid pace, causing both excitement and curiosity among medical professionals, tech enthusiasts, and patients alike. Imagine a world where diseases are diagnosed with precision before symptoms even arise, where treatments are custom-tailored to each individual's genetic makeup, and where recovery times are shortened by predictive insights. AI is laying the groundwork for such possibilities, turning what was once deemed impossible into palpable potential. As we stand on the cusp of this revolution, understanding where we are and where we're going becomes paramount.

With AI's integration into healthcare, we're witnessing a paradigm shift from reactive to proactive care. Diagnostics, once confined to symptom analysis and interpretation, are now aided by algorithms that can parse through vast datasets with unparalleled accuracy. Treatment plans, traditionally based on generalized medical knowledge, are increasingly shifting towards personalization thanks to AI's capability to process and learn from complex biological data. The doctor-patient relationship is evolving, with AI facilitating more informed interactions, allowing for shared decision-making powered by deep insights.

The implications of AI extend far beyond clinical settings. In public health, AI is a powerful tool for disease surveillance, capable of predicting outbreaks and tracking disease progression at a scale and speed unimaginable just a decade ago. In administrative functions, it's streamlining operations, reducing paperwork, and enabling healthcare providers to focus more on patient care. Moreover, the integration of AI in chronic disease management, mental health support, and even telemedicine underscores its versatility and wide-ranging impact.

However, this brave new world isn't without its challenges and questions. With great power comes the responsibility to navigate ethical dilemmas, overcome technological barriers, and ensure equitable access to these advanced tools. As AI becomes more entwined in the healthcare fabric, issues of data privacy, algorithmic bias, and regulatory oversight garner significant attention. It's critical that as we celebrate AI's potential, we also address these concerns thoughtfully and diligently, ensuring technology serves humanity in the most ethical and effective manner possible.

Addressing the ethical considerations and societal implications is as crucial as the technological advancements themselves. Each stakeholder in the healthcare ecosystem—be it a healthcare provider, a patient, a tech developer, or a policymaker—has a role to play in shaping this narrative. Collaborative efforts between these groups will be vital in ensuring AI is developed and implemented in ways that are fair, transparent, and beneficial to all. The conversation around AI in healthcare must be inclusive, engaging voices from diverse backgrounds and perspectives to fully understand and harness the technology's promise.

Looking ahead, the future of AI in healthcare seems boundless. The ongoing research and development in AI not only promise to refine existing medical procedures but also to initiate groundbreaking discoveries. Whether it's through genomic data analysis paving the way for precision medicine, or AI-driven platforms revolutionizing how we approach global health challenges, the scope is vast. The potential for innovation in healthcare that envelopes both advanced urban centers and remote rural areas underscores AI's far-reaching capability to touch every corner of the globe.

This book intends to unravel the layers of AI in healthcare, aimed at a wide array of readers who are committed to exploring these transformative changes. Healthcare professionals, tech innovators, and curious individuals will find insights that shed light on how AI is influencing care delivery, health outcomes, and even roles within the healthcare workforce. By delving into the intersection of technology and medicine, this narrative seeks to not only inform but inspire continued innovation and conversation around the use of AI in healthcare.

The healthcare community stands at an exciting intersection where the fusion of human expertise and machine intelligence can achieve things previously thought unattainable. As you explore the chapters ahead, let the stories and insights serve as a catalyst for understanding the profound impact of AI in healthcare. The journey of AI in medicine is just beginning, and its trajectory holds the promise of a healthier, more informed world.

Chapter 1:
The Rise of Artificial
Intelligence in Medicine

In recent years, artificial intelligence has emerged as a transformative force in the field of medicine, driving unprecedented advancements in how we diagnose, treat, and care for patients. By harnessing the power of complex algorithms and machine learning, AI is not just a tool but a collaborator in the medical field, capable of identifying patterns and insights that often elude human analysis. Healthcare systems are now experiencing a shift from traditional practices to more dynamic, AI-driven approaches, aiding clinicians in making more accurate and personalized decisions for their patients. From detecting intricate subtleties in imaging data to predicting patient outcomes with astonishing precision, AI's integration into medicine is redefining possibilities. This evolution holds promise for not only enhancing the efficiency of healthcare delivery but also democratizing access to high-quality care across patient populations worldwide. As this journey unfolds, ethical considerations and the commitment to maintaining a human touch in medical interactions remain at the forefront, ensuring that technology serves as a complement to, rather than a replacement for, the essential roles of empathy and compassion in healthcare.

The Evolution of AI Technology

Artificial intelligence has not only transformed industries but has also spearheaded a remarkable journey in the realm of medicine. To truly appreciate its impact, it's essential to delve into the evolution of AI technology. The roots of AI trace back to the mid-20th century when the idea of machines simulating human intelligence sparked the imagination of scientists and researchers. In medicine, this evolution has paved the way for revolutionary changes, turning once science-fictional dreams into our modern reality.

Initially, the scope of AI in healthcare was limited by technology and computational constraints. Early computers lacked the immense processing power required to handle the vast quantities of data that AI applications demand. Nevertheless, these humble beginnings laid the groundwork for future innovations. Machine learning, a subset of AI, emerged as a key player—offering the capability to learn from data and improve over time without being explicitly programmed. This learning ability turned AI into a tool that could provide insights far beyond human capacity.

In the 1980s and 1990s, AI's potential in healthcare began to be realized more fully as computational power increased and databases expanded. Expert systems, which simulate the decision-making ability of a human expert, allowed for more sophisticated diagnostics. These systems were primarily rule-based, relying on fixed algorithms, offering only a glimpse of what AI might achieve. Yet, their success underlined a crucial point: AI could significantly aid healthcare professionals by sharing the cognitive load and suggesting possible diagnoses.

The turn of the millennium brought exponential growth in data collection and advancements in computing infrastructure, setting the stage for AI to flourish across industries. In healthcare, these advancements fueled the development of algorithms capable of analyzing complex datasets swiftly and accurately. Deep learning, a form of machine learning based on artificial neural networks, emerged to enable pattern recognition beyond what was previously imagined. Now, AI systems can analyze medical images, predict disease progression, and even suggest treatment plans—a far cry from the static expert systems of the past.

One of the pivotal moments in AI's evolution was the emergence of big data. The sheer volume of information available today allows AI systems to learn with unprecedented depth and accuracy. In healthcare, electronic health records and genomic data provide a treasure trove of information that AI processes to extract actionable insights. Moreover, the integration of AI with wearable technology has brought about a digital health revolution, enabling continuous patient monitoring and real-time health data analysis, thus personalizing patient care like never before.

With the dawn of powerful AI frameworks, such as TensorFlow and PyTorch, the research and development of AI technology have accelerated. These frameworks have democratized AI research, allowing institutions worldwide to contribute to medical innovations. The collaborative nature of this evolution has spurred rapid advancements in personalized medicine, preventive care, and early disease detection. AI is now an indispensable component of research and healthcare delivery systems globally.

The evolution of AI has not been solely a matter of technological progress. It has been shaped by the visionaries and innovators who foresaw AI's potential impact on medicine. Their perseverance in the face of skepticism and technological challenges has propelled AI from concept to reality. The collaboration between technologists and healthcare professionals has been particularly transformative. Together, they have fused domain knowledge with technological expertise, fostering innovations that were once inconceivable.

Nonetheless, AI's evolution continues to face challenges. Ensuring algorithmic transparency and addressing ethical concerns remain pivotal as AI technologies become more integrated into clinical settings. The need for accountability and unbiased decision-making underpins the ongoing development of AI systems. These concerns, though complex, inspire a progressive view of AI—tools that have the potential to empower rather than replace, augmenting human judgment with data-driven precision.

As AI technology continues to evolve, its horizon continually expands. Current research is exploring federated learning, which promises to enhance privacy by decentralized data analysis—a vital exploration in healthcare where patient confidentiality is critical. Quantum computing represents another frontier, promising unprecedented acceleration of AI computations. The interplay between these evolving technologies will likely lead AI into new realms of possibilities, rewriting the boundaries of medicine as we know them.

In summary, the evolution of AI technology marks a period of extraordinary advancement in medicine. This evolution reflects the relentless pursuit of technological and scientific knowledge aimed at improving human health and longevity. By harnessing the power and potential of AI, the medical community is not only enhancing care delivery but redefining the very essence of healthcare itself. The journey of AI in medicine is ongoing, with its future chapters poised to be as impactful as its past: a future where innovation continues to save lives and enrich the human experience.

Key Players in AI and Healthcare

The intersection of artificial intelligence and healthcare is bustling with innovation, driven largely by a diverse group of key players who are shaping this rapidly evolving landscape. These entities range from tech giants with vast resources to nimble startups daring enough to defy traditional norms. Each of these players offers unique contributions to the integration and advancement of AI in healthcare, paving the way for what many believe is a new era of medicine.

Prominent amongst these innovators are the technology behemoths like IBM, Google, and Microsoft. With their significant investment capabilities and technological prowess, they're developing AI solutions that stand at the forefront of healthcare advancements. IBM's Watson, for instance, has been pivotal in proving AI's potential in diagnosing diseases and personalizing treatment plans. Its ability to sift through massive amounts of medical data to find clinically relevant insights is just one example of how AI is being harnessed to improve outcomes.

Google Health, as part of Alphabet, is another major player, leveraging its knowledge in AI and Big Data. They have embarked on ambitious projects like improving healthcare accessibility and early-detection systems using AI. By combing through diverse datasets, their AI-driven efforts aim to provide actionable insights for providers, helping them make informed decisions swiftly and accurately.

Microsoft isn't far behind in this AI-driven healthcare revolution. Through its healthcare division, Microsoft is focusing on cloud-based AI platforms that assist in everything from managing patient data to supporting complex medical research. They've also made strides in developing AI tools that drive collaboration and data sharing across healthcare systems, making treatment more efficient and connected across various entities.

Then, there are startups such as Tempus and PathAI, which are disrupting traditional models by introducing specialized AI innovations. Tempus, for instance, focuses on precision medicine using AI to analyze clinical and molecular data. By integrating AI with genomic sequencing, they strive to tailor treatments more precisely to individual patients' genetic profiles. PathAI, on the other hand, uses AI to enhance pathologists' diagnostic capabilities, promoting error reduction and improving the accuracy of disease detection, especially in complex fields like cancer diagnosis.

The pharmaceutical industry isn't sitting idle, either. Companies such as Pfizer and AstraZeneca are actively integrating AI in drug discovery processes. These giants collaborate with AI-focused firms to accelerate the development of new drugs, enhance the efficiency of clinical trials, and identify promising therapeutic targets that may have previously been overlooked. By leveraging AI, they hope to bring life-saving medications to market quicker and more cost-effectively.

Research institutions and academia are also indispensable players in this ecosystem. Universities and research centers, like Stanford University and the Mayo Clinic, are at the cutting edge of AI research in healthcare. They provide a critical interface between theoretical advances in AI and practical healthcare applications, often forming symbiotic relationships with tech companies to bring innovative solutions to fruition.

Public health organizations are increasingly embracing AI to manage and prevent disease outbreaks. The Centers for Disease Control and Prevention (CDC), for instance, utilizes AI-driven data analytics to better predict and respond to emergent health threats. This predictive capability is invaluable in preparing and responding to pandemics and other large-scale health crises.

Furthermore, non-profits and global health organizations play a critical role in ensuring that AI advancements benefit diverse populations, particularly in underserved areas. Organizations such as the Bill & Melinda Gates Foundation invest in AI technologies that support global health equity. Their initiatives focus on leveraging AI to solve pressing health issues in developing countries, like reducing infant mortality and combating infectious diseases.

Additionally, the role of policy-makers can't be understated in the context of AI in healthcare. Governments worldwide are tasked with crafting regulations that balance innovation with ethics and privacy protection. By setting clear guidelines, they aim to foster an environment where AI can thrive while safeguarding public trust and safety.

Lastly, we must recognize the end-users—healthcare professionals and patients—as key players, too. Their willingness to embrace AI technologies is vital to their successful implementation and continued development. Medical practitioners, for instance, must adapt to AI-enhanced workflows, while patients' acceptance of AI in their care journey is crucial to its widespread adoption.

The synergy among these diverse players—ranging from tech companies and startups to healthcare providers and regulators—creates a dynamic landscape that propels AI-driven healthcare innovations forward. As each player continues to push boundaries and collaborate, the future of medicine is being rewritten in ways that promise better care for individuals and societies alike.

Chapter 2:
AI in Diagnostics

Emerging as a beacon of transformative potential, AI in diagnostics is reshaping the way healthcare professionals approach disease identification. It's not just about speeding up the process; it's about enhancing precision and sensitivity to levels once deemed unattainable. By leveraging complex algorithms and vast data sets, AI empowers practitioners to pinpoint abnormalities with astonishing accuracy, minimizing human error. In clinical settings around the globe, AI-driven tools are already detecting cancers at earlier stages and identifying subtle patterns in genetic and imaging data that were previously invisible to the human eye. This isn't just futuristic speculation—AI tools are actively being integrated into medical workflows, ushering in a new era where diagnostics are not only quicker but more reliable. As AI continues to evolve, its potential to save lives and improve patient outcomes seems boundless, igniting a sense of hope and possibility for the future of medicine.

Enhancing Accuracy in Diagnostics

The dawn of artificial intelligence (AI) in healthcare has ushered in an era where the precision of diagnostics is rapidly evolving. While traditional diagnostic methods have served the medical community for centuries, they've often been fraught with limitations, including variability in interpretation and reliance on subjective judgment. The integration of AI seeks to overcome these hurdles by offering a level of accuracy and objectivity that was previously unattainable.

AI's prowess in diagnostics is primarily rooted in its ability to sift through vast layers of data, spotting patterns that are imperceptible to the human eye. Machine learning models, one of the cornerstones of AI technology, have proven particularly adept at this. These algorithms can analyze complex datasets, such as medical images and genomic data, to identify subtle deviations that might signify the presence of disease. For example, in fields like radiology, AI tools can detect and discern anomalies in imaging studies faster and, in some cases, more accurately than human radiologists, thereby enhancing early detection of conditions such as cancer.

The technology underlying these advancements often involves neural networks, specifically convolutional neural networks (CNNs), which mimic the human brain's processing capabilities. Trained on millions of samples, these networks learn to classify and predict outcomes with staggering efficiency. Thus, they empower healthcare practitioners not only to diagnose illnesses with greater precision but also to predict disease trajectories, potentially revolutionizing prognosis and monitoring.

It's not just in imaging where AI shines. In pathology, AI systems are used to digitize slides, enabling detailed analysis that can enhance diagnostic accuracy and consistency. These systems analyze the cellular morphology at a granular level, offering insights that lead to more precise classifications of diseases. AI holds promise in reducing diagnostic errors, which can occur when human limitations are tested by fatigue or cognitive biases.

Moreover, AI's contribution to diagnostics extends beyond the individual patient. Population health advances through large-scale epidemiological studies have uncovered patterns that inform public health initiatives. By analyzing extensive datasets from various populations, AI algorithms can detect outbreaks earlier and with more specificity, guiding policy interventions and resource allocation.

This unprecedented accuracy doesn't come without challenges. Integrating AI into diagnostic procedures necessitates substantial investment in technology and training. Medical professionals must be adept at understanding AI outputs to leverage them effectively. The shift requires rethinking traditional roles within healthcare, where the doctor's eye and the machine's precision collaborate for the best outcomes.

Ethically, there's a pressing need to ensure that AI systems are trained on diverse datasets to avoid biases that could lead to inaccurate diagnoses in underrepresented groups. Transparent algorithms and equitable access to AI-driven diagnostics are critical to ensuring that advancements benefit all segments of the population, not just those in technologically advanced regions.

A particularly transformative aspect is AI's potential to customize diagnostic approaches for personalized patient care. In personalized health, AI can tailor diagnostic techniques based on individual health profiles, which improves specificity and sensitivity. For instance, AI can integrate a patient's genetic information, lifestyle, and environmental factors, providing a thorough basis for risk assessment and early intervention.

The merging of AI with genomics is driving breakthroughs in diagnostics for genetic disorders. Algorithms process genomic sequences with remarkable speed, highlighting variants that could indicate a predisposition to certain conditions. The ability to rapidly interpret genetic data is poised to assist in diagnosing rare diseases, often riddled with diagnostic delays, thereby impacting treatment timelines and patient outcomes favorably.

AI's enhancement of diagnostic accuracy is proving inspirational to healthcare professionals who see their roles changing from mere diagnosticians to strategic partners in patient management. By freeing clinicians from routine tasks attributed to diagnostics, AI allows them to focus more on developing therapeutic relationships with patients and devising personalized treatment strategies.

The role of AI in diagnostics presents an opportunity to revisit and refine our understanding of medicine itself. As diagnostic tools become more sophisticated, there's a continuous push towards improving existing algorithms and creating more robust datasets that encompass diverse patient demographics. The hope is that as AI systems advance, they will learn beyond individual diseases to understand the broader biological underpinnings of health and disease, potentially preventing illness before it starts.

In conclusion, enhancing accuracy in diagnostics through AI is not just about improving specific techniques; it is about forging a new path in medicine that leverages technology for holistic patient care. While challenges remain, the opportunities AI presents have the potential to redefine diagnostics, serving as the pinnacle of innovation in modern healthcare. The journey has just begun, and its impact on the landscape of diagnostics is bound to be profound and lasting. As we progress, the possibilities are not just limited to what AI can do but extend to how it can deepen our understanding of health in ever more meaningful ways.

Real-World Applications of Diagnostic AI

As artificial intelligence increasingly intertwines with the field of diagnostics, its real-world applications have grown both in scope and impact. Diagnostic AI is transforming the healthcare landscape by enhancing the accuracy and efficiency with which medical conditions are identified and assessed. From advanced imaging techniques to the analysis of vast datasets, AI is solving complex problems that were previously beyond our reach. These innovations aren't just theoretical; they're actively shaping the way clinicians approach diagnosis in hospitals, clinics, and even in remote care settings.

One of the most profound applications of diagnostic AI lies in imaging, particularly in radiology and pathology. AI tools that analyze medical images can identify patterns and anomalies with greater precision than ever before. For instance, deep learning algorithms are trained to detect tumors in digital mammograms and can often highlight subtle indicators that a human might miss. The consistent unveiling of such hidden details aids radiologists in making more informed decisions, potentially catching diseases at their most treatable stages.

Pathology, too, benefits significantly from AI's capabilities. Machines trained on large datasets can analyze biopsy samples, identifying cancerous cells with a level of accuracy unattainable by the naked eye. This kind of diagnostic support can ensure that patients receive timely and accurate treatments, ultimately improving their prognosis. Moreover, the ability of AI to learn and adapt means that its performance only improves with time, resulting in diagnostic standards that continue to rise.

Besides traditional imaging and pathology, AI is making waves in genomics. The analysis of genetic data is often a daunting task due to its sheer volume and complexity. AI-driven tools can sift through genomic information, identifying mutations and genetic markers associated with various conditions. Such insights are crucial not just for diagnostics but for the broader field of personalized medicine, where tailored health interventions can be devised based on an individual's genetic profile.

AI also standardizes diagnostic practices across the board, reducing discrepancies that might arise from human error or subjective interpretation. This uniformity ensures that no matter where a patient is located or which physician they consult, they receive a diagnosis that relies on the same high-level benchmarks. This aspect is especially valuable in rural or under-resourced areas where expert consultation may be limited or delayed. AI can bridge these gaps, providing a level of diagnostic precision previously only available in well-equipped urban centers.

Beyond improving accuracy, AI in diagnostics is speeding up the diagnostic process itself. By automating certain routine analyses, AI frees medical professionals to focus on more complex cases that require human intuition or experience. In emergency situations, where every second counts, quick and precise diagnostics can mean the difference between life and death. AI is providing the tools necessary for rapid triaging and treatment initiation, thereby saving lives and optimizing resource use.

Real-world applications of diagnostic AI are not confined to physical ailments. Mental health is another critical area where these technologies are being harnessed. AI-based applications have been developed to analyze speech patterns, sleep data, and even social media activity to predict and diagnose mental health disorders such as depression and anxiety. This ability to monitor and potentially diagnose from everyday activities offers a non-invasive way to identify individuals at risk and facilitate early intervention.

Moreover, through wearable technology and mobile apps, AI is bringing diagnostic capabilities directly to patients. These tools can monitor vital signs, track chronic conditions, and even alert healthcare providers in case of irregularities. The implication is a more proactive approach to health management, where patients are more engaged and healthcare becomes a continuing dialogue rather than periodic check-ins.

In the field of infectious diseases, AI has shown exceptional promise in early detection and response. Algorithms capable of tracking patterns in public health data can detect outbreaks and even predict their trajectory. They can process real-time data from across the globe, offering a level of detail that enables health organizations to respond swiftly and effectively. AI's capability to model the spread of infectious diseases helps in implementing timely countermeasures, which is particularly crucial in densely populated or resource-limited areas.

Despite these countless benefits, it's vital to approach AI in diagnostics with careful consideration. The integration of artificial intelligence into healthcare systems requires thorough validation to ensure reliability and safety. Data security and patient privacy remain crucial, and AI's role should always complement the expertise of healthcare professionals rather than replace it.

Diagnostic AI is not just about machines taking over tasks; it's fundamentally about enhancing human capabilities and reshaping healthcare into a more predictive, efficient, and precise practice. As AI technology continues to evolve, its applications in diagnostics will undoubtedly grow, potentially uncovering new insights into diseases and offering innovative ways to enhance human health. The future holds promise for a more profound collaboration between AI and healthcare professionals, driven by a common goal: improving patient outcomes and advancing medical science in unprecedented ways.

Chapter 3:
AI-Driven Treatments

As artificial intelligence continues to evolve, it's transforming the landscape of medical treatments by making them more personalized, precise, and proactive. No longer confined to the realm of diagnostics alone, AI is now an invaluable ally in the development of individualized treatment plans that cater to the specific genetic makeup and lifestyle factors of each patient. This innovative approach not only improves the effectiveness of treatments but also reduces the possibility of adverse effects, offering a level of customization previously unimaginable. Success stories abound as AI systems analyze vast quantities of data to uncover unique patterns and correlations, leading to breakthroughs in disease management and therapy effectiveness. By harnessing machine learning algorithms and predictive analytics, healthcare providers can make more informed decisions, ultimately enhancing patient outcomes. As we navigate this frontier, the merger of AI and medicine promises a future where treatments are not just reactive, but anticipatory, aligning perfectly with the aspirations of precision medicine.

Personalized Medicine through AI

At the heart of the revolution in modern medicine lies the potential of personalized medicine—a vision that tailors treatment to the individual characteristics of each patient. Artificial intelligence (AI) is pivotal in making this vision a reality. By analyzing vast and complex datasets, AI enables healthcare providers to create more effective, patient-specific treatment plans. Traditional medicine often relies on a one-size-fits-all approach, which can overlook the unique aspects of each patient's condition. AI disrupts this model by considering various factors such as genetics, lifestyle, and environment, ensuring that treatments are not only personalized but also predictive and preventive.

Understanding how AI facilitates personalized medicine begins with genetic data. Modern AI algorithms can analyze large-scale genomic information with remarkable efficiency, uncovering insights that were previously unattainable. This capability allows for the identification of genetic markers associated with certain diseases, providing clinicians with the knowledge to develop targeted therapies. For example, AI has been used to predict how different patients will respond to chemotherapy, even before treatment begins. Such predictive modeling can spare patients from unnecessary side effects and optimize therapeutic outcomes.

The scope of personalized medicine powered by AI extends well beyond genomics. AI systems are adept at integrating multifaceted data ranging from electronic health records to real-time sensor data from wearable devices. This integration forms a comprehensive picture of patient health, enabling precise interventions. Consider cardiovascular care, where AI analyzes data from wearable heart monitors to detect anomalies that might indicate an impending cardiac event. This real-time analysis empowers patients and physicians to take proactive measures, potentially averting a major health crisis.

Moreover, AI doesn't merely assist in treatment personalization; it radically transforms drug development. Traditional drug discovery is a lengthy and costly process, often taking years to develop a single drug. AI streamlines this process significantly by predicting how different compounds might interact with target receptors in the body, identifying promising drug candidates faster. Personalized medicine benefits tremendously from this advancement, as AI algorithms can match patients with drugs tailored to their specific genetic makeup and health profile, leading to higher efficacy and lower risk of adverse reactions.

One of the most motivational aspects of AI-driven personalized medicine is its potential to democratize healthcare. By making sophisticated analyses accessible, AI lowers the barriers for resource-constrained environments to implement advanced medical strategies. For instance, in regions with limited access to endocrinologists, AI can facilitate personalized diabetes management by continually analyzing blood sugar levels and adjusting insulin doses accordingly. This reduces dependency on constant expert supervision, empowering patients to manage their condition more independently.

Ethical considerations are integral to the conversation surrounding personalized medicine through AI. As systems access and process sensitive patient data, concerns around privacy and security inevitably arise. Ensuring data is anonymized and securely stored is crucial for maintaining patient trust and compliance with regulations. Ethical AI also involves transparency in how personalized recommendations are made, allowing patients to understand and consent to AI-based interventions confidently. Collaborative efforts among tech developers, healthcare professionals, and policymakers are essential to navigate these ethical landscapes effectively.

Despite the challenges, AI has already paved the way for remarkable success stories in personalized medicine. Cancer treatment has experienced significant breakthroughs, with AI systems aiding in the identification of unique tumor characteristics, leading to individualized immunotherapy treatments that enhance survival rates. Similarly, rare diseases, which often receive less research attention, benefit from AI's ability to pool global data, identifying treatment possibilities based on patterns discovered across diverse case studies.

The journey toward personalized medicine through AI is an ongoing narrative of innovation and collaboration. As AI technologies evolve, so too does their capacity to deliver nuanced insights that shape patient-centric approaches. Crucial to this evolution is the relentless pursuit of cross-disciplinary research, integrating expertise from fields such as bioinformatics, machine learning, and clinical medicine. This integration fosters a robust framework where AI not only meets but anticipates the diverse needs of patients.

It is inspiring to envision a future where AI-driven personalized medicine is not an alternative but the norm. Imagining a world where each individual's healthcare journey is mapped out with precision and empathy, guided by data that speaks to their unique biological makeup, inspires hope for vastly improved outcomes. Undoubtedly, the intersection of AI and personalized medicine is redefining what it means to be treated as a whole person, rather than just a set of symptoms, ushering in an era of healthcare where precision meets personalization.

Success Stories in AI Treatment

In the era where data and technology converge to transform healthcare, AI has emerged as a beacon of hope, reshaping the landscape of medical treatment. Its integration into patient care marks a significant leap forward, demonstrating possibilities that were once confined to the realm of science fiction. Through a blend of computational power and clinical insight, AI has achieved feats that resonate with both awe and inspiration, illustrating its profound impact with real-world success stories.

Consider the story of Emma, a young girl diagnosed with a rare form of leukemia. Traditional treatment regimens had limited success, leaving her family in a state of despair. Enter Watson, IBM's AI-driven platform. By analyzing vast datasets from medical literature and patient records in mere minutes, Watson pinpointed a personalized treatment plan, offering a pathway that conventional methods hadn't identified. Emma's condition improved remarkably, demonstrating the potential AI holds in tailoring precision treatments that hinge on individual genetic and health profiles.

In another compelling narrative, AI proved itself indispensable in the field of neurology. A hospital faced challenges with stroke patients, particularly in the rapid assessment needed to decide when and if a clot-busting drug should be administered. The decision-making window was perilously narrow, and delays could mean the difference between life and a lifetime of disability. By deploying an AI system specifically designed to analyze brain scans swiftly and with high accuracy, the hospital reduced decision times significantly. This not only saved lives but also improved patient outcomes substantially, showcasing the synergistic potential of AI where time equals neurons.

There's also the intriguing case of diabetic retinopathy, a leading cause of blindness worldwide. Health clinics in under-resourced regions often lack the skilled professionals needed to diagnose early stages of this condition. AI-based tools, such as Google's DeepMind, have stepped in to fill this gap. These AI systems can analyze retinal scans with more accuracy than their human counterparts, detecting signs of disease long before symptoms manifest. Such advancements in diagnostics push boundaries, ensuring that even in remote locales, patients are afforded the same quality of care as those in tech-enabled urban hospitals.

Oncology, the study and treatment of tumors, stands among the frontlines where AI is making remarkable strides. Treatment plans are complex and multifaceted, often involving a delicate balance of chemotherapy, radiation, and surgery. AI algorithms support oncologists by providing insights into the likely efficacy of various treatment combinations based on historical data from thousands of similar cases. As a result, these tailored interventions maximize patient comfort and minimize side effects, paving the way for improved quality of life during treatment engagements.

In the realm of mental health, AI has broken new ground by offering innovative interventions for conditions like depression and anxiety. Applications using natural language processing algorithms can evaluate subtle nuances in speech and writing, indicators often too subtle for human therapists to catch early. These AI tools complement traditional therapeutic sessions by providing real-time insights and recommendations, facilitating more proactive mental health interventions. For many, this means earlier support and better management of their mental health challenges, illuminating a path towards long-term well-being and recovery.

The landscape of chronic disease management also benefits deeply from AI innovations. One success story involves chronic obstructive pulmonary disease (COPD), where AI-driven applications monitor patient symptoms and environmental conditions. By collecting and analyzing comprehensive real-time data, these systems predict flare-ups before they happen. Patients, thus, gain a proactive strategy, adjusting their medication or lifestyle accordingly to prevent hospital admissions, which are both costly and life-disruptive.

It's crucial to illustrate the impact of AI through these lived experiences and measurable improvements in patient care. The success stories serve not just as a testament to technological prowess but as a reminder of the empathetic dimension AI can bring to medicine. By focusing on personalization—tailoring treatments and interventions to individual needs—AI is aligning itself as an ally, perhaps even a savior, especially in scenarios where conventional methods fall short.

Moreover, the adaptability of AI treatment methods enhances patient engagement. Apps and tools foster a participatory health model, encouraging patients to take ownership of their health journey. Interactions with these tools are intuitive, often designed to simulate an empathetic human connection, which inspires confidence and adherence to treatment plans. This dynamism ensures that AI's application isn't just reactive but continuously evolving, factoring in patient feedback and emerging health trends.

These success stories underscore the potential of AI to not only augment clinical decisions but transform them. By redefining the architecture of treatment modalities across multiple disciplines, AI is expanding the horizons of what's possible in healthcare, fueled by both statistical certainty and human empathy. As these stories continue to unfold, they advance a narrative of hope and progress, forging a path towards a future where technology and compassion harmoniously coexist.

Looking ahead, the possibilities are boundless. As AI continues to learn and evolve, it promises to unlock further potential in areas that remain challenging in contemporary healthcare. Collaboration between AI developers, healthcare professionals, and policymakers is crucial in translating this potential to every corner of the global health landscape. It's an endeavor charged with the promise of success that bears witness to its profoundly transformative power.

AI's stories of success, therefore, are not just about technological feats. They're about people: patients whose lives have been touched, families whose burdens have been eased, and communities that stand to benefit from an equitable healthcare future. With every case, every success, and every life enhanced, AI advances its deep-rooted commitment to healing and hope.

Chapter 4:
AI in Surgery

A I in surgery is transforming the operating room into a realm where precision meets innovation, propelling surgical practices into a groundbreaking future. Imagine surgeons working hand-in-hand with intelligent robots, where AI not only assists with complex surgical tasks but also enhances the surgeon's capability to make critical decisions in real-time. This revolutionary partnership isn't just about increasing the accuracy of procedures but also aims to reduce recovery times and improve patient outcomes significantly. With advanced imaging and data analytics, AI empowers surgeons to anticipate complications before they arise, crafting a new standard for operational success. As AI continues to evolve, it's clear that the fusion of human expertise with machine intelligence heralds an era where the impossible in surgery becomes achievable, inspiring medical professionals and benefiting patients worldwide.

Robotics and Surgical Precision

In the realm of surgery, precision is not just preferred; it is paramount. The advent of robotic systems integrated with artificial intelligence (AI) has heralded a new era in achieving unparalleled precision in surgical procedures. Robotics in surgery isn't exactly brand new, but the integration with AI systems has acquired remarkable momentum recently. These advancements are characterized by increased accuracy, minimized tissue damage, and more rapid patient recovery times.

One of the colossal strengths AI brings to robotic surgery is its ability to enhance the surgeon's dexterity and visualization. Imagine conducting a delicate procedure deep within the body's cavities with minimal invasion. With AI-enabled robots, surgeons can translate fine wrist movements into precise mechanical motions. These mechanical limbs don't suffer from fatigue, nor are they prone to human error. Equipped with machine learning algorithms, they can continuously improve performance, creating a feedback loop that optimizes surgical outcomes.

Robotic systems like the da Vinci Surgical System have paved the way for AI integration by marrying the intuitive movements of a surgeon with computer-enhanced precision. This synergy has been transformative in minimally invasive surgeries, such as prostatectomies and cardiac valve repair. Surgeons, who may once have struggled with the spatial restrictions of traditional surgery, now operate through tiny incisions, dramatically reducing blood loss and recovery time.

AI's role isn't limited to mechanical precision. It extends to planning and decision-making. Advanced AI algorithms analyze preoperative imagery and data to suggest optimal surgical paths and strategies. For example, in brain surgery, exact navigation is crucial. AI can process MRI scans to create a 3D model of the patient's brain, mapping out the safest and most effective path to the target area while avoiding critical neural pathways.

Let's consider the feedback mechanism embedded in AI-driven robotic systems. These systems are equipped with haptic feedback, a tactile response technology allowing surgeons to 'feel' the texture and resistance of tissues from afar. Such technology provides surgeons an extra layer of sensory information, and potential errors are identified before they cause any harm. This capability fosters a unique blend of human intuition and machine reliability.

In addition to enhancing physical precision, AI empowers robotic systems to become partners in the surgical decision-making process. Algorithms can use data from countless similar surgeries to recommend approaches and warn about potential complications, turning data into real-time, actionable insights. This democratizes surgical proficiency, potentially benefitting surgeons who have less experience in complex procedures with the expertise of seasoned specialists reflected through intelligent systems.

But the journey doesn't stop here. The evolution of AI in robotics is ongoing and multifaceted. Researchers are exploring the incorporation of AI-driven analytics and big data to track long-term outcomes of robotic surgeries. This data can be invaluable in fine-tuning procedures and customizing them according to individual patient needs, enabling a shift towards truly personalized surgical care.

The ethical considerations surrounding AI-powered robotic surgery merit attention as well. As these systems gain autonomy, questions regarding accountability arise. Who is responsible in the event of a malfunction or error — the developers, the manufacturers, or the surgeons operating these systems? Such questions demand careful examination and highlight the need for robust regulatory frameworks.

Moreover, AI in robotic surgery has the potential to address global healthcare disparities. Rural or underserved areas can benefit from AI-assisted tele-surgery, opening access to expert surgical intervention regardless of geographical constraints. While the infrastructure for widespread use is still being established, the possibilities for global health equity are optimistic and inspiring.

Despite these advancements, one should not view AI and robotics as replacements for skilled surgeons but as enablers that enhance human capability. The human element remains irreplaceable, vital for critical decision-making, empathetic patient interaction, and ethical judgment. The confluence of human expertise with robotic precision heralds a future where surgeries are safer, more efficient, and profoundly effective.

In conclusion, the integration of AI in robotic surgery signifies more than a technological leap; it's a paradigm shift in how we envision surgical care. Through enhanced precision and elevated decision-making capabilities, AI's partnership with robotics carries immense potential to revolutionize the field, providing benefits that resonate far beyond the operating table. We stand on the cusp of this transformative change, with AI-driven surgical precision poised to define the future landscape of global healthcare. The intersection of robotics and AI in surgery doesn't just promise better outcomes; it heralds a future where surgical excellence is within reach, redefining what's possible in medicine today.

AI-Assisted Procedures

In the world of surgery, precision and efficiency are paramount. Surgeons constantly seek ways to enhance their capabilities while minimizing risks and improving patient outcomes. AI-assisted procedures stand at the forefront of this evolution, offering unprecedented support that transforms the surgical landscape. By integrating artificial intelligence into surgical practices, we're witnessing a shift from purely human-dependent operations to a synergistic relationship where AI augments human expertise.

Central to AI-assisted surgeries is the deployment of advanced robotics that work in tandem with surgeons. These robotic systems, powered by AI, not only improve precision but also reduce the likelihood of human error. For example, in minimally invasive surgeries, AI-driven robots can be programmed to make incredibly accurate movements that even the steadiest human hands might struggle to match. This level of control opens new possibilities for procedures that require extreme delicacy, such as neurosurgery, where millimeter-level accuracy can make all the difference.

But AI's contribution doesn't end at physical assistance. AI algorithms are becoming crucial in pre-operative planning and intra-operative decision-making. These algorithms can analyze vast amounts of patient data, including medical history, imaging results, and genetic information, to provide insights that help tailor surgical procedures to each individual's unique needs. As a result, surgeons are better equipped to anticipate complications and make informed decisions before and during surgery, which leads to improved patient safety and recovery outcomes.

This integration also extends to enhancing visibility during operations. AI systems, utilizing machine learning and computer vision, can interpret real-time surgical footage to identify and highlight critical anatomical structures, ensuring that surgeons have the most accurate information available as they work. This capability is particularly valuable in complex procedures, where identifying and avoiding key structures can mean the difference between success and complications.

Moreover, AI-assisted procedures are democratizing surgery by leveling the playing field for less experienced surgeons or those at the beginning of their careers. Through machine learning, AI systems can be trained on thousands of previous surgical cases, learning best practices and common pitfalls. These systems can then offer recommendations or warnings in real-time, effectively acting as a mentor that provides guidance during the procedure. In this way, AI not only boosts the capabilities of expert surgeons but also empowers those in training, accelerating their journey toward proficiency.

Looking beyond the operating room, the data collected during AI-assisted surgeries have significant implications for surgical education and research. By analyzing this data, researchers can identify trends and correlations that were previously invisible. This newfound knowledge can help refine surgical techniques, develop new procedures, and create training modules that ensure future surgeons are armed with the best possible information.

AI is also helping break down geographical barriers in surgical care. Through telepresence and robotic-assisted surgeries, expert surgeons can perform or guide procedures from half a world away. This possibility means that patients in remote or under-resourced locations can access world-class surgical care without the need to travel. AI provides the precision and assistance needed to conduct these complex procedures remotely, ensuring the quality of care is maintained.

Despite all these advancements, the rise of AI-assisted procedures brings new challenges and considerations. Ethical issues surrounding autonomy and the potential for over-reliance on AI are significant. It's crucial that the integration of AI doesn't diminish the essential human touch and judgment that characterize the art of surgery. Professional integrity and ongoing oversight must remain at the heart of surgical practices to ensure AI is a tool that complements, rather than supplants, the human element.

Furthermore, the implementation of AI-assisted technologies requires significant investment in infrastructure, training, and maintenance. Hospitals and surgical centers must prioritize the continuous education of their teams to keep pace with rapid technological advancements. This investment is not just financial but also an investment in creating an adaptable surgical workforce that embraces these new tools and techniques.

In conclusion, AI-assisted procedures represent a transformative milestone in the field of surgery. By blending AI's data-driven precision with human experience and intuition, surgery is reaching new heights of effectiveness and safety. As these technologies continue to evolve, they promise to revolutionize the surgical landscape, making high-quality care more accessible and personalized than ever before. The key to harnessing AI's full potential will be continued collaboration among technologists, medical professionals, and policymakers to ensure these innovations are integrated ethically and equitably into healthcare systems worldwide.

Chapter 5:
AI in Radiology

The integration of AI in radiology is profoundly transforming how imaging techniques are approached, analyzed, and applied. Radiologists are now harnessing the power of AI algorithms to enhance image interpretation, significantly improving the speed and accuracy of diagnoses. This transformative shift allows for a level of precision in identifying abnormalities that was previously unattainable, heralding a new era in diagnostic radiology. Not only does AI assist in identifying subtle patterns that may escape the human eye, but it also provides predictive insights that support clinicians in delivering personalized patient care. These advancements are proving invaluable, particularly in early disease detection, where timely intervention can dramatically alter patient outcomes. As AI continues to evolve, radiologists are learning to adapt and incorporate these tools into their practice, leading to collaborative environments where technology and human experience work hand in hand. This synergy holds the promise of elevating the entire field to new heights, ensuring that patients receive the most accurate and timely diagnoses possible, paving the way for more individualized treatment plans.

Transforming Imaging Techniques

As artificial intelligence (AI) continues to revolutionize radiology, one area undergoing significant transformation is imaging techniques. Radiology has always been a cornerstone of modern medicine, providing a window into the human body through various imaging modalities. AI is supercharging this process, enhancing the capability, accuracy, and efficiency of imaging practices.

AI's influence on radiological imaging begins with its ability to process vast amounts of data quickly and accurately. Traditional imaging techniques, while advanced, come with the limitation of human error. Radiologists face challenges such as fatigue and information overload, particularly with the increasing complexity of imaging data. AI algorithms, specifically designed to handle such issues, offer the potential to interpret images with less subjectivity and error, thereby improving diagnostic accuracy.

Imagine AI as a digital assistant for radiologists, rapidly identifying patterns and anomalies that might elude the human eye amidst numerous images. Deep learning, a subset of AI, has shown great promise in recognizing specific conditions within medical images. For instance, it can detect minute changes in tissue that might suggest the early onset of diseases like cancer. This capability is pivotal in enabling early and potentially life-saving interventions.

Incorporating AI into imaging techniques is also transforming the workflow within radiology departments. By automating routine tasks, AI frees radiologists to focus on more complex aspects of diagnostic interpretation and patient interaction. Automated image analysis reduces the turnaround time for reports, thus leading to quicker, more efficient patient management. This forms a crucial part of a healthcare ecosystem increasingly leaning towards precision medicine.

Another exciting aspect of AI in transforming imaging techniques is its capability to enhance image quality. Noise reduction algorithms, empowered by AI, make it possible to obtain clearer images at lower radiation doses in modalities like CT scans without losing diagnostic quality. This is especially beneficial for vulnerable populations, such as children, who need to minimize radiation exposure.

Through advanced techniques like image reconstruction, AI is changing how radiologists view and manipulate images. AI can synthesize high-resolution images from lower-quality datasets, giving clinicians improved visuals for analysis and diagnosis without subjecting patients to additional or repeated scans. This transformation is not just about doing things faster; it's about doing things smarter.

Virtual reality (VR) and augmented reality (AR), in conjunction with AI, are pushing imaging visualization into new dimensions. These technologies provide radiologists with immersive 3D models generated from two-dimensional image data, offering new perspectives and insights impossible with standard imaging. The integration of such technologies is particularly beneficial in complex surgical planning or when explaining medical conditions to patients.

Furthermore, AI continually learns and improves from each interaction. Machine learning models refine their predictive accuracy over time as they are exposed to more data and confirmed diagnoses. This ongoing learning process leads to continuous improvement in the reliability of AI-assisted imaging interpretations, ultimately contributing to better patient outcomes and reduced healthcare costs.

Ethical practice and quality assurance are essential when AI is integrated into medical imaging. It is crucial that these models are rigorously validated and consistently reviewed by radiologists to ensure that AI complements human expertise rather than replaces it. The symbiotic relationship between AI and human professionals is at the heart of transforming imaging techniques, ensuring the highest standards in patient care.

As we look toward the horizon, AI promises further advancements in imaging, including personalized imaging protocols based on a patient's genetic and physiological profiles. Future imaging techniques might automatically adjust settings to optimize the balance between image quality and exposure risks for individual patients. Personalized imaging heralds a new era of truly individualized medicine, where AI tailors diagnostics and treatments to each person's unique characteristics.

In conclusion, AI is reshaping radiological imaging, driving improvements in accuracy, efficiency, and personalization. Harnessing AI's computational power and pattern recognition capabilities enables earlier diagnosis, refined imaging techniques, and enhanced patient experience in radiology. The transformation of imaging techniques through AI is not just a technological evolution but a step towards a more intelligent and empathetic healthcare system.

Case Studies in AI-Radiology Integration

Artificial intelligence has woven itself into the fabric of radiology, offering new vistas of possibility in diagnostics and patient care. In this section, we will explore the remarkable integration of AI into radiology through real-world case studies that underscore its transformative potential. These examples are not merely technological triumphs; they are narratives of progress that illustrate how AI is redefining the capabilities of radiology departments worldwide.

One of the most compelling case studies comes from the United Kingdom, where the National Health Service (NHS) has implemented an AI system to aid in the early detection of breast cancer. Utilizing deep learning algorithms, this AI tool analyzes mammograms with a precision that rivals human radiologists. What sets this initiative apart is its dual focus on accuracy and accessibility. By streamlining the diagnostic process, the NHS aims to reduce waiting times and ensure that more patients receive timely interventions. Initial reports reveal a significant decline in the rate of false negatives, a critical improvement that can translate into life-saving early treatments for many women.

Across the Atlantic, the University of California, San Francisco (UCSF), has pioneered a novel application of AI in the interpretation of chest X-rays. Their system employs an AI algorithm known as CheXNet, which is specifically designed to identify signs of pneumonia. CheXNet's training involved processing over 100,000 X-ray images to develop its ability to recognize pneumonia better than expert radiologists. The implications extend beyond mere diagnostic accuracy; this development promises to alleviate the workload on radiologists, speed up diagnosis in emergency settings, and ultimately enhance patient outcomes by enabling quicker clinical decisions.

Meanwhile, in India, an AI-driven initiative aims to transform tuberculosis (TB) diagnosis. This project leverages AI to automate the analysis of X-rays, assisting in the identification of TB, particularly in rural areas where specialist radiologists are scarce. This AI system operates even on low-quality images, a common issue in resource-limited settings. The success of this initiative hinges on its ability to bridge the gap in healthcare infrastructure, offering a glimpse of how AI can democratize healthcare by making advanced diagnostics available to underserved populations.

On the technological frontier, Stanford University's AI lab has been at the forefront of developing AI tools that challenge traditional diagnostic frameworks. By employing machine learning algorithms, they have introduced models that can predict the progression of neurodegenerative diseases through brain imaging. These tools provide insights into brain structures over time, offering a quantitative assessment that was previously infeasible with conventional imaging techniques. With the ability to assess changes at a microscopic level, this approach holds the promise of revolutionizing the way diseases like Alzheimer's are diagnosed and monitored.

In commercial applications, several tech giants have entered the arena with AI solutions tailored for radiology. One such initiative involves the collaboration between Google Health and a prominent London hospital chain to enhance the detection of head and neck cancer via AI. By employing their vast computational resources, these AI models rapidly process complex imaging, offering detailed analyses that assist radiologists in identifying malignancies at earlier and more treatable stages. This partnership exemplifies how AI can augment the human element in radiology, combining computational power with clinical expertise to yield better patient outcomes.

Exploring the successes and challenges of AI in radiology wouldn't be complete without considering the role of regulatory bodies. For instance, the FDA's rapid approval of AI software in imaging diagnostics highlights the evolving landscape of medical regulations. By emphasizing safety and efficacy, regulatory bodies play a crucial role in ensuring that AI applications enhance patient care without compromising accuracy or reliability. This interplay between innovation and regulation ensures that as AI systems continue to evolve, they do so within frameworks that prioritize patient safety and ethical standards.

At the heart of these advancements lies a profound shift in how radiologists interact with technology. Traditionally, radiology has been a practice deeply rooted in the keen observational skills of expert practitioners. With the advent of AI, these skills are now being augmented with computational prowess, creating a symbiotic relationship that expands the possibilities of what can be achieved within a radiology department. AI doesn't replace the human element; instead, it enhances radiologists' ability to interpret complex data and focus their expertise on cases that require nuanced judgment.

While these case studies illustrate promising advancements, they also highlight challenges that health professionals and technologists must navigate. Integrating AI into radiology involves not only technological implementation but also a cultural shift within medical communities. Training and education are essential for radiologists to harness AI's full potential effectively. Institutions worldwide are currently working towards integrating AI training into radiology education to ensure future radiologists are equipped with the tools they need to work alongside AI seamlessly.

The journey of AI integration in radiology is iterative, requiring constant refinement and an openness to novel methodologies. It also necessitates collaboration across disciplines—from data scientists and engineers to medical professionals and ethicists—to drive forward the innovation that ultimately enriches patient care. As AI continues to extend its reach, the field of radiology stands at the cusp of further breakthroughs that are set to redefine healthcare paradigms.

In summary, these case studies exemplify how AI is being harnessed to tackle some of the most pressing challenges in radiology, paving the way for more efficient, accurate, and accessible diagnostic tools. Each story represents a step towards a future where AI's partnership with radiology not only enhances diagnostic capabilities but also bridges gaps in healthcare delivery across the globe. The potential for AI in radiology is immense, beckoning a future where technology continues to push the boundaries of what medicine can achieve.

Chapter 6:
AI and Drug Discovery

In the realm of drug discovery, artificial intelligence is working wonders, transforming what was once a lengthy and costly process into a more efficient journey from lab to patient care. Researchers now leverage advanced algorithms to analyze vast datasets, identifying potential drug candidates with remarkable speed and precision. This acceleration isn't just a technological feat; it's a gateway to curing diseases more swiftly and effectively. AI-driven models predict how compounds interact at a molecular level, uncovering promising therapeutic paths that may have been overlooked by traditional methods. The collaborative power of AI and pharmacology is not only energizing the pharmaceutical industry but is also providing hope with innovations that promise to address unmet medical needs. As AI continues to evolve, it sets the stage for a future where life-saving treatments are developed faster and more accurately, reshaping drug discovery for the betterment of global health.

Accelerating Drug Development

The path of drug development has traditionally been a long and arduous journey, often spanning over a decade from initial discovery to regulatory approval. However, with the advent of artificial intelligence, this process is undergoing a significant transformation. AI's ability to process vast amounts of biological data and identify promising drug candidates is reshaping how pharmaceuticals are developed, cutting down the time and costs traditionally associated with this endeavor.

AI's prowess lies in its capacity to quickly analyze and interpret complex biological data. By sifting through genomic data, protein structures, and potential drug interactions, AI algorithms can identify potential drug targets in a fraction of the time it would take human researchers. This ability not only accelerates the pace of drug discovery but also enhances precision, potentially leading to more effective and safer drugs.

One of the key advantages of AI in drug development is its capacity to perform what is known as in silico drug testing. Traditional drug testing methods often involve a significant amount of time and resources spent on laboratory testing. In contrast, in silico approaches use computational models and simulations to predict how a drug might interact with biological systems. This ability can significantly reduce the need for preliminary laboratory tests, expediting the transition from discovery to clinical trials.

Beyond early-stage discovery, AI also plays a crucial role in optimizing clinical trials. AI can identify suitable candidates for trials more efficiently by analyzing patient data, such as genetic information and electronic health records. This targeted approach not only accelerates trial recruitment but also enhances the accuracy of trial outcomes by ensuring a more appropriate match between drug and patient. Moreover, AI algorithms can monitor trial data in real-time, identifying trends and results swiftly, thus potentially speeding up the decision-making processes related to trial continuation or modification.

The integration of machine learning techniques into drug development processes isn't just theoretical—it's already bearing fruit. For instance, several biotech companies have leveraged AI to develop promising drug candidates in oncology and neurology at unprecedented speeds. One notable example is the rapid identification of potential drug candidates during the COVID-19 pandemic, where AI models helped screen thousands of compounds to narrow down those most likely to succeed in clinical settings within months rather than years.

AI isn't only revolutionizing the speed of drug development but also its creativity. Traditional research methodologies may often follow familiar pathways dictated by prior knowledge and experience. However, AI approaches can lead to the discovery of unconventional molecules and methods, opening doors to innovative therapeutic avenues previously unexplored due to limitations in human bias and computational power.

The potential of AI-driven drug development extends globally, promising to have a particularly significant impact on neglected diseases that have historically suffered from underfunding and lack of research due to the limited commercial viability for pharmaceutical companies. With AI reducing costs and resource demands, the development of drugs for such diseases becomes more feasible, potentially leading to breakthroughs where they are desperately needed.

Collaboration is at the heart of AI's success in drug development. It brings together experts from the fields of computer science, biology, chemistry, and medicine to work on emerging technologies and datasets. This multidisciplinary approach fosters innovation and ensures that AI tools are continuously refined to meet the complexities of biological systems, allowing for more accurate and meaningful analyses.

The ethical considerations in AI-driven drug development are not negligible. While the technology offers numerous advantages, it also presents challenges, particularly regarding data privacy and the potential for algorithmic bias. Ensuring that patient data is handled responsibly and algorithms are transparent and fair remains a crucial component of the ongoing deployment and acceptance of AI in this field.

As we look toward the future, the acceleration of drug development through AI promises not just a streamlined process but one that is densely packed with potential for medical breakthroughs. The speed and efficiency offered by AI mean that the gap between research and patient benefit may soon be significantly reduced. This potential to bring life-saving drugs to market rapidly could transform treatment landscapes for various diseases, offering hope where little previously existed.

In conclusion, AI is not just a tool but a transformative force in drug development, revolutionizing the timeline, cost, and creativity of pharmaceutical research. By continuing to harness the capabilities of AI, we stand on the brink of a new era in medicine—one where drug development is more responsive, adaptable, and ultimately more aligned with the urgent health needs of the global population.

Innovations in AI-Driven Pharmacology

In recent years, artificial intelligence has surged to the forefront of pharmacology, marking a pivotal shift in how drugs are discovered and developed. This transformation is not merely a technological upgrade but a fundamental rethinking of drug discovery processes. Gone are the days when drug development relied heavily on the slow and labor-intensive trial-and-error methods. Today, with AI's computational prowess, our approach to pharmacology has evolved into a more predictive and efficient enterprise.

One of the most compelling innovations involves the use of AI to model biological systems. By simulating the interactions between drug candidates and biological pathways, AI systems can predict therapeutic outcomes with a higher degree of accuracy than traditional methods.

This modeling capacity enables researchers to understand complex biological mechanisms, leading to the identification of potential drug targets that were previously overlooked. With AI, the drug development journey begins on a solid scientific foundation, enhancing the likelihood of successful outcomes.

AI's ability to analyze massive datasets rapidly and accurately is revolutionizing how pharmaceutical researchers handle and interpret experimental data. Advanced machine learning algorithms sift through high-throughput screening results, genomic data, and electronic health records to identify promising drug candidates. These algorithms can uncover patterns and correlations across datasets, revealing insights that might go unnoticed by human analysts. This capacity for deep data analysis accelerates the discovery of novel drugs and repurposes existing medications for new therapeutic applications, thereby reducing time-to-market and cost.

Furthermore, AI excels at predicting drug toxicity and side effects, a challenge that has long plagued pharmacology. Traditional methods often discover such issues late in development, sometimes resulting in costly failures. AI algorithms, however, can predict adverse reactions early by analyzing chemical structures and historical data from similar compounds. This predictive power not only minimizes risks but also ensures that only the safest drug candidates proceed to clinical trials, safeguarding patient health and conserving resources.

In clinical trials, AI-driven tools are proving invaluable for patient stratification and personalized medicine. By using genetic information and other biomarkers, AI can identify subgroups of patients likely to respond favorably to a particular treatment. This precision reduces trial sizes and durations, thus making clinical trials more efficient and ethically sound, and increasing the likelihood of regulatory approval.

The integration of AI into clinical decision support systems represents another innovation, particularly in adaptive trial designs.

These AI systems optimize clinical trial parameters in real-time based on incoming data, allowing for seamless adjustments to study protocols. As a result, pharmaceutical companies can make informed decisions quickly, improving the probability of trial success while adapting to new insights as they arise.

The rise of automated synthesis platforms driven by AI highlights a remarkable trend in pharmacology—machines that suggest and test novel compounds autonomously. With minimal human intervention, these AI systems conduct chemical experiments, evaluate results, and refine their hypotheses, iterating towards optimal solutions at a pace unachievable by human researchers. This autonomous exploration underscores AI's potential to expand the drug development arsenal significantly.

Moreover, AI's role in optimizing drug manufacturing processes cannot be overstated. Predictive maintenance driven by AI ensures that production lines operate smoothly, predicting machine failures before they occur and reducing downtime. Enhanced process control mechanisms improve product quality and consistency, ensuring that patients receive medications that meet rigorous standards.

A noteworthy development is the collaboration between AI and other advanced technologies, such as quantum computing. While still nascent, this synergy promises exponential improvements in computational chemistry, drug optimization, and complex problem-solving. By leveraging quantum computing's prowess in tackling large-scale combinatorial problems, AI can refine drug candidates faster, honing in on the best molecular structures for therapeutic use.

In the quest for personalized medicine, AI stands at the cutting edge. By integrating genetic, environmental, and lifestyle data, AI systems tailor drug regimens to individual patient profiles. This approach promises treatments that are more effective, with fewer side effects, fulfilling the long-held dream of personalized pharmacotherapy. Through continuous learning, AI systems evolve over time, refining their predictions and treatment recommendations, thus delivering customized healthcare solutions that align with each patient's unique needs.

Despite these promising advances, the implementation of AI in drug discovery is not without challenges. Ethical considerations, such as data privacy and algorithmic bias, remain critical concerns that must be addressed to ensure equitable access to AI-enhanced treatments. As we embrace these innovations, it is crucial to maintain transparency and build trust among stakeholders, including patients, healthcare providers, and regulatory agencies.

The unfolding narrative of AI-driven pharmacology is one of progress and possibility. It offers a glimpse into a future where drug development is faster, safer, and more attuned to the nuances of human biology. By marrying AI's computational strengths with the intellectual rigor of pharmacological science, we are crafting a new era in medicine—one where the impossible becomes possible, and where science fiction evolves into scientific reality.

As we stand on the brink of this transformative era, the prospects for improved healthcare are truly inspiring. Through global collaborations and multidisciplinary efforts, AI-driven pharmacology is not just a theoretical construct but a practical, life-changing force. It challenges the limits of our imagination and encourages us to envision a world where diseases are not merely managed but fundamentally understood and overcome.

Chapter 7:
AI in Patient Care

As healthcare continuously evolves, artificial intelligence is increasingly becoming an integral part of patient care, transforming how we monitor and manage health on an individualized basis. AI platforms are revolutionizing the process by providing real-time patient data, enabling care teams to make informed decisions promptly. Through advanced algorithms, AI offers predictive analytics that anticipate patient needs, thereby reducing the risk of complications and enhancing overall outcomes. Consider AI as a diligent assistant that learns patterns and adapts swiftly to each patient's unique conditions and responses. This inspiring capability fosters a more proactive and personalized approach to medicine, bridging gaps between patient interaction and professional practice. By leveraging AI, healthcare providers are not just treating patients; they're envisioning the future of wellness with tools that envelop empathy and precision, a testimony to technology's potential in reshaping patient care paradigms. With AI's footprint growing in medical environments, we witness a blend of innovation and compassion in healthcare like never before.

Monitoring and Managing Patient Health

Monitoring and managing patient health has always been a complex orchestration of observation, data collection, and interpretation. Technological advancements are now pushing the boundaries further by introducing artificial intelligence into this critical facet of healthcare. AI's role in this area is both profound and transformative. It's no longer about simply collecting data; it's about understanding and interpreting it to enhance patient wellbeing in real-time and beyond.

At the heart of this transformation is the development of wearables and smart devices, which have become integral in monitoring patient health. These devices collect vast amounts of data from patients, tracking everything from heart rates to activity levels. The data collected is then processed by AI algorithms that can identify patterns and anomalies with speed and precision that humans can't achieve alone. This ability to continuously monitor health metrics allows for the detection of potential health issues before they become critical.

One of the remarkable aspects of AI in patient monitoring is its capability for predictive analytics. For patients with chronic conditions like diabetes or heart disease, AI can analyze historical data to predict future health events. This predictive ability empowers patients and healthcare providers to engage in proactive care management, potentially reducing hospitalizations and improving quality of life.

It's important to note, however, that this technology isn't limited to chronic conditions alone. AI is making waves in acute care settings as well. For example, smart sensors in hospital beds can monitor vital signs and body movements, alerting staff to potential complications like bed sores or falls. These advancements exemplify AI's potential to enhance patient care environments, ensuring both safety and responsiveness.

An interesting development in this field is the enhancement of personalized healthcare plans. By leveraging AI, healthcare providers can create bespoke treatment and monitoring strategies tailored to individual patient needs. This customization is achieved through the sophisticated data analysis capabilities of AI, which can synthesize information from various sources such as patient history, genetic information, lifestyle data, and more. The result is a healthcare plan that is not only reactive but also anticipatory.

The integration of AI into patient monitoring isn't solely about technology; it's about collaboration between humans and machines. AI doesn't replace healthcare professionals; rather, it augments their capabilities. It allows providers to shift their focus from routine data collection and monitoring tasks to more critical decision-making and patient interaction. This synergy has the potential to drive more empathetic and effective patient care.

Nevertheless, the deployment of AI in monitoring and managing patient health does pose certain challenges. Privacy concerns and data security are at the forefront, given the sensitive nature of health information. The massive amounts of data generated require robust security measures to prevent breaches and ensure patient confidentiality. Moreover, there's a need for clear regulatory frameworks to guide the ethical use and storage of data.

In terms of system integration, healthcare providers face the challenge of incorporating new AI systems into existing healthcare infrastructures. Interoperability is vital for these technologies to deliver their full potential. Ensuring that various devices and systems can communicate seamlessly is crucial in creating a cohesive and efficient monitoring network.

Data interpretation is another area that demands attention. While AI systems are impressive in pattern recognition and data analysis, the nuances of human health are sometimes beyond the scope of programmed algorithms. The collaboration between AI and healthcare professionals is key in interpreting these data accurately, balancing technological insights with human intuition and experience.

Looking to the future, AI-driven patient monitoring systems are poised to become even more sophisticated with advancements in machine learning and data analytics. With the continuous influx of new data and the refinement of AI algorithms, these systems will not only monitor but also engage in continuous learning. This evolution promises to push the boundaries of predictive analytics and precision medicine even further, making healthcare more proactive and patient-centric.

The role of AI in monitoring and managing patient health is a testament to how technology can transform healthcare. By enhancing our understanding of patient health, AI systems empower both patients and providers in the pursuit of improved health outcomes and greater autonomy over healthcare decisions. As these technologies evolve, they hold the promise of transforming not only patient monitoring but the entire healthcare paradigm, potentially redefining how we understand and approach health management in profoundly innovative ways.

AI Platforms for Improved Care

In the evolving landscape of healthcare, AI platforms are not just tools—they're transformative allies. As technology creeps further into every corner of patient care, AI platforms have emerged as powerful enablers of improved care delivery. These platforms seamlessly integrate with existing systems to augment human capabilities, offering a new frontier where medical professionals can push beyond traditional boundaries.

From managing complex patient schedules to predicting potential health crises days in advance, AI platforms are a boon for healthcare providers. They eliminate inefficiencies, streamline operations, and allow staff to focus on the most important aspect of healthcare—patient interaction. Through comprehensive data analysis, these platforms offer insights that were once unimaginable. They don't just compile data; they translate it into actionable plans that can prevent disease and manage chronic conditions more effectively.

A pivotal role of AI platforms is in predictive analytics. These sophisticated systems can sift through vast amounts of historical patient data and demographic-specific health records to predict impending health events. Hospitals and clinics, armed with this data, can manage their workflows and resources more effectively. For instance, predicting patient influx during flu season allows healthcare facilities to allocate resources efficiently, ensuring they are prepared well in advance.

Furthermore, AI platforms are redefining patient engagement. By leveraging natural language processing and advanced algorithms, these systems can interact with patients through chatbots and virtual assistants. They provide 24/7 support, answer queries, schedule appointments, and remind patients about medication and upcoming health checkups. This constant engagement not only ensures adherence to treatment plans but also builds a strong doctor-patient relationship, vital for positive health outcomes.

Implementing robust AI platforms facilitates personalized care plans that are tailored to each patient's unique needs. By assessing individual patient data, including genetic predispositions and lifestyle factors, these systems propose personalized interventions. Such precision medicine approaches are not only more effective but also help in minimizing potential adverse effects of generalized treatment protocols.

In addition, AI platforms support care teams in making better clinical decisions by offering evidence-based recommendations. These systems quickly analyze new studies, clinical trials, and medical records in relation to a current case, delivering valuable insights that inform diagnostic and treatment choices. Medical professionals can thereby focus on their critical thinking and judgment skills, rather than spending precious hours sifting through mountains of research papers.

Operational efficiency is another area where AI platforms make a significant impact. Administrative tasks like billing, coding, and scheduling can be prone to human error; however, with AI's intervention, these processes become streamlined and largely error-free. Automated systems can also ensure compliance with regulations and facilitate smooth accreditation processes, offering peace of mind in an otherwise high-pressure environment.

Moreover, AI platforms enhance the monitoring and management of patient health beyond the hospital walls. With the integration of wearable technologies and IoT devices, real-time health data is fed back to care teams, allowing them to monitor vitals and make timely interventions. This real-time data-sharing capability enables proactive care, reduces emergency hospitalizations, and supports a model that prioritizes keeping patients healthy rather than just treating illness.

Despite their potential, the implementation of AI platforms is not without challenges. There's the need for robust infrastructure, data privacy concerns, and the necessity of integrating these platforms with legacy systems. Overcoming these hurdles involves collaboration between tech developers, healthcare providers, and policymakers to ensure that these platforms are both effective and secure.

AI platforms have started transforming healthcare at a fundamental level. From enabling precision medicine and supporting clinical decisions to enhancing patient engagement and streamlining operations, these systems offer a glimpse into the future of healthcare—one that's efficient, personalized, and compassionate. We've only just begun to understand the scope of what AI can achieve in improving care, and the journey ahead promises to be revolutionary in shaping better health outcomes for all.

Chapter 8:
AI in Chronic Disease Management

In the realm of chronic disease management, artificial intelligence emerges as a beacon of hope, reshaping how we approach long-term health conditions like diabetes and cardiovascular disease. AI technologies are empowering healthcare professionals to offer more personalized and efficient care plans by leveraging vast amounts of data from patient histories and real-time monitoring tools. Imagine AI algorithms predicting a diabetic patient's glucose fluctuations with remarkable accuracy or anticipating potential heart issues before they become critical, allowing timely interventions. Such advancements not only enhance the quality of life for patients but also reduce the burden on healthcare systems by minimizing hospital admissions and complications. Moreover, AI-driven applications enable patients to participate actively in their health management through user-friendly platforms that provide insightful feedback on lifestyle changes. The fusion of AI with chronic disease management symbolizes a transformative shift towards a more proactive, preventative approach in healthcare, where intelligent systems work alongside medical professionals to impact lives profoundly and positively.

Applications in Diabetes Management

In recent years, the management of diabetes has undergone a remarkable transformation, driven largely by the integration of artificial intelligence (AI) technologies. As one of the most prevalent chronic diseases worldwide, diabetes poses significant challenges both to individual patients and to healthcare systems. AI offers promise in addressing these challenges through innovations in monitoring, treatment, and lifestyle management.

One of the most impactful applications of AI in diabetes management is in the realm of continuous glucose monitoring (CGM). AI algorithms are able to analyze glucose data in real time, providing insights that can predict glucose trends and alert patients to potential hypoglycemic events before they occur. This predictive capability allows for proactive management, reducing emergency situations and improving overall quality of life.

AI also enhances the management of diabetes through its ability to personalize treatment plans. By taking into account a variety of factors such as genetics, lifestyle, and daily routines, AI systems can tailor medication and dietary recommendations to fit individual needs. This has paved the way for more precise insulin dosing, crucial for maintaining optimal blood glucose levels, especially for those with type 1 diabetes.

Moreover, AI platforms often integrate with wearable technology, empowering patients with real-time feedback and coaching on lifestyle choices. Smart devices, such as fitness trackers and smartwatches, can monitor physical activity, dietary intake, and even stress levels, providing a holistic view of a patient's health. The AI then synthesizes this data, offering suggestions that encourage healthier habits, which are vital for diabetes management.

Another groundbreaking application of AI in diabetes is in the early detection and prevention of disease-related complications. Diabetic retinopathy, a leading cause of blindness in diabetes patients, can now be detected early through AI-assisted retinal imaging. Algorithms trained to identify minute changes in retinal images can alert healthcare providers to intervene promptly, preventing significant vision loss.

Furthermore, in the realm of clinical decision support, AI models analyze large datasets from diverse patient populations to uncover patterns that might not be apparent to human clinicians. This capability aids in stratifying patients based on risk and tailoring interventions accordingly, whether they involve lifestyle modifications or pharmacological treatments. The aim is to prevent the progression of diabetes and mitigate associated health risks.

The integration of AI in diabetes management extends to addressing disparities in care as well. By leveraging AI-driven telehealth platforms, patients in remote or underserved areas gain access to specialized diabetes management resources. These platforms facilitate ongoing communication between patients and their healthcare team, ensuring that treatment plans are adapted as necessary and that patients don't fall through the cracks.

AI also plays a vital role in research and development, accelerating the pace at which new treatments and technologies are evaluated. Machine learning models can analyze clinical trial data to identify promising trends and predict outcomes, expediting the transition from research to practice. This not only fosters innovation but also ensures that patients benefit from the latest advancements in diabetes care at a faster rate.

In terms of patient education, AI technologies can equip individuals with actionable insights and personalized learning materials tailored to their level of understanding and specific needs. Virtual coaching systems, for example, utilize conversational AI to engage patients in interactive sessions about diabetes management skills, reinforcing their confidence and ability to self-manage their condition effectively.

Nevertheless, while the potential applications of AI in diabetes management are vast and transformative, it's essential to address the challenges they introduce. Ensuring the privacy and security of patient data is paramount, given the sensitive nature of health information. Moreover, the effectiveness of AI systems hinges on the quality of data they're trained on—raising concerns about algorithmic bias and the need for inclusive datasets.

It's crucial, too, for healthcare providers to remain at the helm, using AI as a supplement rather than a replacement for their expertise. By blending AI innovations with the empathetic touch of human care, the future of diabetes management holds promise for more intuitive, effective, and equitable solutions.

In summary, AI's impact on diabetes management is profound, offering innovative tools that equip patients and clinicians with greater control over the disease. From predictive monitoring and personalized treatment to enhanced education and research acceleration, AI not only empowers proactive management but also paves the way for breakthroughs in care delivery. As these technologies continue to mature and evolve, they promise to redefine the landscape of diabetes management, heralding a new era in chronic disease care.

AI Tools for Cardiovascular Health

Artificial intelligence has found fertile ground in the arena of cardiovascular health. With cardiovascular diseases being the leading cause of death globally, the need for effective and efficient management strategies is undeniable. AI tools have stepped into this critical space, offering a fresh approach to prediction, prevention, and treatment that was unthinkable just a decade ago. AI's role here isn't simply futuristic; it's already affecting real-world outcomes, transforming how healthcare professionals handle one of the most pressing health challenges of our time.

Perhaps one of the most promising aspects of AI in cardiovascular care is its potential to predict heart attacks before they happen. Traditional risk assessment methods rely heavily on factors such as age, cholesterol levels, and blood pressure. However, AI systems can analyze vast datasets to identify patterns that may not be obvious to the human eye. This capability significantly enhances the accuracy of predictions. For example, machine learning algorithms trained on millions of patient records can now discern subtle heart irregularities in ECG data that might signal an impending heart attack.

The integration of AI into wearable technology is another frontier making significant strides in cardiovascular health management. Devices like smartwatches are now more sophisticated, equipped with sensors that continuously track heart rates and other vital signs. AI processes this continuous stream of data, detecting anomalies instantly. These wearables don't just serve as early warning systems; they empower individuals to take an active role in their health management, offering a blend of convenience and life-saving potential.

AI-driven platforms that specialize in cardiovascular imaging are also revolutionizing diagnostics. Cardiac imaging, including MRI and CT scans, provides detailed pictures of the heart and vessels. AI algorithms sift through these images to identify conditions like plaque build-up, heart muscle abnormalities, and congenital heart disease. The speed and accuracy with which AI can process these images often outpace traditional methods, which can be slow and expensive. This means quicker diagnoses and more timely treatments for patients.

Consider also the role of AI in personalized treatment plans. Cardiovascular conditions often require highly individualized strategies that take into account the patient's unique risk factors and lifestyle. AI tools analyze data from a range of sources, including genetic information, patient history, and even socioeconomic factors, to recommend treatment options that are tailored specifically to the individual. Such precision medicine approaches enhance treatment efficacy and patient satisfaction, minimizing the trial-and-error aspect of conventional treatments.

Beyond prediction and diagnostic imaging, AI plays a substantial role in monitoring chronic cardiovascular conditions. Systems such as AI-enhanced telehealth platforms allow healthcare providers to remotely monitor heart patients regularly. These systems can spot signs of deterioration early, ensuring that interventions can be made before a patient requires emergency care. In doing so, telehealth reduces the burden on healthcare systems and provides patients with a degree of independence and flexibility unimaginable a few years ago.

Moreover, AI-enhanced robotic systems are increasingly used in interventional cardiac procedures. In catheterization labs, AI aids in everything from positioning to the actual movement of instruments within delicate vessels. This enhances precision and reduces the risk of human error, improving outcomes for patients undergoing complex procedures like angioplasties or valve repairs.

Data analytics, a cornerstone of AI, offers insights that would otherwise remain hidden in mountains of cardiovascular research. AI algorithms can parse through studies with thousands of participants, identifying correlations and causal relationships that increase our understanding of heart disease mechanisms. This continuous feedback loop between AI and research fuels ongoing innovations in heart health management.

Ethical considerations still loom large over the widespread implementation of AI in cardiovascular health. The potential for bias in algorithms that learn from historical data cannot be ignored, especially in diverse populations with varying risk profiles. It's crucial that developers and healthcare providers work in tandem to ensure that AI tools are equitable and accessible to all patients, thereby truly transforming cardiovascular care across the board.

The role of AI in cardiovascular health stands as a testament to the remarkable and evolving capabilities of technology in medicine. These tools are more than just upgrades to existing practices; they represent a paradigm shift. As AI continues to delve deeper into the intricacies of heart health, the horizon grows more promising, offering a glimpse of a future where cardiovascular diseases can be predicted, prevented, and treated with unprecedented precision and care.

Chapter 9:
AI in Mental Health

In the realm of mental health, artificial intelligence is emerging as a game changer, bringing transformative innovations to how we identify and treat mental disorders. With the growing prevalence of mental health issues, AI offers promising tools that promise timely intervention, from sophisticated algorithms analyzing patterns to predict susceptibility to mental illnesses, to virtual therapists providing around-the-clock support. These AI solutions not only enhance diagnosis accuracy by learning from vast datasets but also extend empathy through AI compassion, bridging the traditional empathy gap in medical technology. This blend of technology and care offers a more accessible and personalized approach to mental health treatment, encouraging a new era where mental well-being is prioritized and managed with greater precision and understanding. As AI continues to evolve, it holds the potential to revolutionize mental health care in ways we are only beginning to realize, offering hope and support to countless individuals worldwide.

Identifying and Treating Mental Disorders

In the realm of mental health, artificial intelligence is paving new pathways for understanding, identifying, and treating mental disorders. The complex nature of mental health issues, combined with the stigma surrounding them, has traditionally posed significant challenges for healthcare providers. However, AI is stepping in as a transformative force, offering innovative solutions that promise to revolutionize the field.

One of the most promising aspects of AI in mental health is its ability to enhance early detection of mental disorders. AI-powered diagnostic tools can analyze a wide array of data — from patient history and electronic health records to social media behavior and wearable technology metrics — to identify patterns indicative of mental health issues. These tools provide clinicians with a more comprehensive view, enabling earlier interventions that can significantly alter the course of a mental illness.

Machine learning algorithms are central to these advancements, as they are designed to improve their accuracy over time by learning from vast datasets. By analyzing subtle cues like variations in speech patterns, facial expressions, and even typing dynamics, AI systems can detect early signs of disorders such as depression and anxiety with remarkable precision. These insights often surpass human capability, as many such signals are too nuanced or complex for clinicians to detect unaided.

Furthermore, AI tools are not confined to well-structured data only. Natural language processing (NLP) allows for the analysis of unstructured data, which includes textual inputs from therapy sessions or personal journal entries. This capability is a breakthrough in assessing the mental state of patients, as it allows AI to interpret language nuances, emotional tone, and the sentiment of patients' expressed thoughts and feelings.

Beyond diagnostics, AI plays a significant role in the treatment of mental disorders. Virtual therapy platforms, powered by AI, are becoming increasingly sophisticated, providing an accessible and scalable means of delivering mental health care. These platforms can engage users in therapeutic conversations, offering cognitive behavioral therapy and mindfulness exercises tailored to individual needs. The advantage is the availability of immediate support, which can be crucial for patients in distress.

AI-driven treatment interventions also include personalized treatment plans. These plans are based on algorithms that assess treatment effectiveness over time, allowing for dynamic and adaptive interventions that are tailored to the individual patient. Such customized approaches increase the likelihood of successful outcomes, as they consider the patient's unique response to different therapies and medications.

In addition, AI is being used to create predictive models which foresee mental health trends within a population. These models help identify at-risk individuals, enabling preemptive measures. For instance, in workplace settings, AI can analyze employee behavior patterns to predict burnout risk, prompting interventions before serious effects manifest.

The utilization of AI in mental health care also holds the potential to bridge the empathy gap often present in traditional clinical settings. While it may seem counterintuitive, AI platforms are being designed to simulate empathetic responses, helping patients feel understood and supported. This capability is especially beneficial in scenarios where human clinicians may lack empathy or cultural understanding.

Ethical considerations are paramount in the integration of AI in mental health care. Privacy concerns, consent, and the potential for algorithmic bias must be carefully managed. The sensitivity of mental health data requires stringent security measures to ensure patient confidentiality. Additionally, ethical frameworks must guide these innovations to prevent misuse and ensure that AI tools are used equitably across diverse populations.

Moreover, the role of human oversight in AI-driven mental healthcare cannot be underestimated. AI should augment, not replace, human clinicians, providing them with additional insights and tools to enhance patient care. Collaboration between technology developers, clinicians, and mental health professionals is essential to ensure that AI systems are safe, effective, and aligned with clinical best practices.

In conclusion, as AI continues to evolve, its potential for transforming mental healthcare grows increasingly apparent. By enhancing diagnostic accuracy, personalizing treatments, and offering novel therapeutic solutions, AI is helping to address some of the most pressing challenges in mental health today. By continuing to refine these technologies and adhere to ethical guidelines, we can unlock their full potential and ensure that AI serves as a compassionate, effective ally in the journey towards better mental health care for all.

AI Compassion: Bridging the Empathy Gap

Artificial Intelligence (AI) in mental health care is a topic that invites both awe and skepticism. On one hand, AI holds the promise of transforming treatment paradigms with its unparalleled data-processing capabilities; on the other hand, there is apprehension about whether technology can truly understand the nuanced human experience of emotional and psychological distress. At the heart of this debate lies a fundamental question: Can AI ever bridge the empathy gap to provide compassionate mental health care?

Compassion is often viewed as a peculiarly human trait, deeply connected to our ability to relate and respond to the emotions of others. It's something that's not only learned but felt, a complex interplay of empathy, understanding, and action. As AI continues to evolve, researchers are exploring if it can emulate, or at the very least, effectively simulate these human characteristics in meaningful ways.

Several breakthrough AI applications in mental health suggest that machines are beginning to inch closer to this elusive goal. AI algorithms can analyze speech patterns, monitor facial expressions, and even detect changes in social media behaviors, offering insights into an individual's mental state. These tools are instrumental in identifying early signs of mental disorders, facilitating timely interventions that might have been missed by human eyes alone.

Yet, technology alone can't capture the essence of human emotion. Machines may recognize the signs of depression or anxiety through data input, but understanding the unique context of each individual's experience is something else entirely. Here, the collaboration between AI and mental health professionals becomes crucial. While AI can handle the heavy lifting in data analysis, it's the mental health specialists who bring in the emotional intelligence to interpret these data in the context of personal histories and lived experiences.

The integration of AI into mental health services is not about replacing therapists and counselors. Instead, it aims to augment their ability to deliver care by offering a more accurate and holistic view of a patient's psychological landscape. This integration allows mental health professionals to focus on the human element of care, using AI insights to better understand and empathize with patients. It's a symbiotic relationship that leverages the strengths of both AI and human intuition.

Innovative AI-driven platforms are already making strides in providing mental health support. Mobile apps using AI can offer therapeutic exercises and cognitive behavioral techniques, providing valuable support between therapy sessions. These platforms can engage users in virtual conversations designed to mimic human-like interaction, offering comfort and guidance. However, it's crucial to ensure that while AI offers support, it doesn't inadvertently increase feelings of isolation by replacing genuine human contact.

Ethical considerations play a significant role in deploying AI in mental health. The privacy of sensitive mental health data, the potential for algorithmic bias, and the transparency of AI processes are all critical concerns that need to be addressed. To bridge the empathy gap, AI systems must not only be technologically robust but also designed with moral integrity at their core. Building trust in AI systems is essential for both patients and practitioners to feel confident in their use.

The challenge remains to create AI systems that are not only capable of understanding data but are also built with fairness and compassion at their core. Researchers are exploring methods to introduce bias-awareness into AI algorithms, enhancing their ability to provide fair and unbiased support across diverse demographic groups. Transparency in AI decision-making processes is another critical step toward building this trust.

Furthermore, ongoing education and communication about the capabilities and limitations of AI in mental health care are important in fostering public trust. Effective collaboration between technology developers, mental health practitioners, and ethicists can help ensure that AI systems are developed responsibly and aligned with the needs of those they aim to serve.

As technology continues to evolve, so too does the potential for AI to play a compassionate role in mental health care. The challenge—and opportunity—lies in ensuring that AI complements the human touch, using its analytical power to support rather than supplant the nuanced, empathetic interactions that define quality mental health care. By doing so, AI can bridge the empathy gap, not by mimicking human emotion, but by enhancing our ability to understand and support emotional well-being through data-driven insights.

AI's journey towards bridging the empathy gap in mental health is ongoing. It reflects broader societal questions about the role of technology in our lives. While AI continues to grow in capability, mental health care professionals will have to navigate this complex landscape thoughtfully and empathetically. Together, they can create a future where technology and human compassion work hand in hand, providing a fuller, richer approach to mental health care. In doing so, they honor both the science and the art of this deeply human field.

Chapter 10:
AI in Genomics

A I has fundamentally transformed genomics, ushering in an era of unprecedented discovery and personalized medical solutions. Through the power of machine learning algorithms, researchers can now decode the vast expanse of genomic data with remarkable speed and precision, uncovering insights that once seemed unimaginable. By parsing through this complex data, AI not only identifies genetic predispositions but also guides the development of targeted therapies tailored to individual genetic profiles. This synergy between AI and genomics is redefining our understanding of genetic diseases and is on the frontier of personalized medicine—a relentless pursuit to tailor treatments uniquely for each patient. The implications are vast, promising not just smarter healthcare solutions but also a journey into the depths of human genetics that holds the keys to many of tomorrow's medical breakthroughs.

Decoding Genomic Data

In the vast and intricate symphony of biological processes, genomic data plays the foundational melody. It is the blueprint of life, dictating everything from our susceptibility to certain diseases to the nuances of personal traits. Yet, interpreting this complex data is no simple task. Enter artificial intelligence—it offers a transformative lens through which we can decode and understand genomics at unprecedented scales. AI in genomics heralds a new age in precision medicine by employing cutting-edge algorithms to disentangle the genetic code.

Genomic data is massive and complex. One person's genome comprises approximately three billion base pairs, the building blocks of DNA. Analyzing such extensive information isn't only resource-intensive but also prone to errors if done manually. AI steps in as a powerful ally, able to sift through vast amounts of data swiftly and with remarkable accuracy. It unravels patterns and correlations, uncovering insights that were previously cloaked in complexity. These capabilities enable breakthroughs not just in genetic research but directly impact patient care by identifying potential genetic predispositions.

Pioneering AI algorithms in genomics have revolutionized how genetic diseases are identified and analyzed. For instance, machine learning applications can predict inherited disorders by comparing genetic sequences against a vast database of known mutations. Speed here is crucial. What once took scientists weeks to decipher can now be achieved in mere hours using AI models. These rapid analyses provide timely and crucial interventions, especially in cases involving genetic disorders that require early treatment to prevent severe outcomes.

Moreover, AI's prowess in pattern recognition allows researchers to identify subtle genetic variations that might be overlooked by traditional methods. These variations, known as single nucleotide polymorphisms (SNPs), can be critical markers of disease. Identifying such markers is essential for early detection and management of complex disorders, like cancer or cardiovascular diseases. Beyond disease prediction, AI is adept at assisting in uncovering the genetic basis for response to therapies, guiding more personalized and effective treatments for individuals.

The use of AI in genomics extends to pharmacogenomics—how a person's genetic makeup influences their reaction to drugs. By understanding these individual variations, AI can help tailor medication dosages, reducing adverse drug reactions and increasing therapeutic efficacy. This application not only boosts patient outcomes but also streamlines operations within the healthcare system, potentially reducing costs associated with trial-and-error prescriptions.

AI also provides a promising frontier for rare disease research. Many of these diseases are tied to specific genetic abnormalities, yet they evade quick detection due to their rarity. AI can trawl through extensive datasets to pinpoint these anomalies with greater speed and precision than human analysis alone. By accelerating the discovery of rare genetic variants, AI not merely expedites patient diagnosis but sparks new avenues for treatment development.

The potential of AI in genomics isn't confined to direct healthcare implications. It also invigorates biomedical research, inviting collaborations that cross geographical and disciplinary boundaries. By sharing anonymized genomic data, researchers globally can collaborate more effectively, pooling AI-driven insights to enhance our collective understanding of genetics. These initiatives propel forward the current understanding of genomics, incrementally building a more comprehensive picture of genetic influences on health and disease.

Ethically, the integration of AI in genomics presents challenges we must navigate. Data privacy is a significant issue. Genetic information, being deeply personal, must be treated with utmost confidentiality. This calls for robust algorithms that not only analyze effectively but also secure data against unauthorized access. Additionally, while AI offers tremendous potential, ensuring that algorithms are free of biases and functional across diverse populations remains critical. Aligning AI's capabilities with ethical practices is imperative for gaining public trust and widespread acceptance of these revolutionary technologies.

The trajectory of AI in decoding genomic data is an exhilarating journey into the unknown, filled with promise and challenges. With

The

continued advancements in AI technology and a growing understanding of its applications, we stand on the cusp of revolutionizing medicine as we know it. As these tools become increasingly integrated into the fabric of healthcare, they hold the promise to reshape diagnostics, prognostics, and therapeutic interventions, mapping a path toward precision medicine where treatments are as unique as the individuals receiving them.

In sum, AI not only acts as a decoder of genomic data but as a catalyst for innovation in healthcare. By unlocking the secrets of our genetic code, it heralds a future where medical treatment is proactive, personalized, and optimally effective. As we refine these technologies and address the ethical considerations they present, we move closer to realizing the full potential of AI in genomics—charting a new realm where the possibilities for better health outcomes are boundless.

Personalized Genomics with AI

In an era defined by technological revolutions, the fusion of artificial intelligence and genomics epitomizes a groundbreaking shift that holds the potential to redefine the landscape of healthcare profoundly. Personalized genomics, powered by AI, is not just an advancement; it's a transformation that tailors medical care by delving into the unique genomic makeup of individuals. This innovative approach offers not only new insights into our genetic frameworks but also paves the way for dramatically enhanced treatment options and preventive care.

By leveraging vast datasets of genomic information, AI systems can identify patterns and correlations that were previously unimaginable. These algorithms can sift through myriad sequences to discern meaningful connections, enabling healthcare providers to craft therapies that are highly individualized. Imagine a world where broad-spectrum treatment plans give way to specialized regimens that account for an individual's genetic predisposition—AI is bringing us closer to that reality.

The personalization of medicine begins with a detailed analysis of the human genome. Sequencing of the genome provides a treasure trove of data that AI can analyze. AI models excel at recognizing complex patterns in this data, facilitating the identification of genetic variants associated with specific health risks. With these insights, practitioners can devise health strategies that not only treat current conditions but also anticipate future issues, allowing for earlier intervention and improved outcomes.

One of the most exhilarating applications of AI in personalized genomics lies in predicting disease susceptibility. Through pattern recognition and machine learning, AI systems are able to identify genetic markers that signify the likelihood of developing conditions such as cancer, heart disease, and more. This empowers patients with the knowledge to make informed decisions about their healthcare, from lifestyle modifications to monitoring plans that preempt the onset of illness. Such proactive approaches can dramatically alter the course of a patient's life.

Beyond disease prediction, AI-driven genomics is transforming how we approach treatment plans. Pharmacogenomics explores how genes affect a person's response to drugs, and with AI's ability to analyze genetic data, we can now customize prescriptions to the individual. This not only improves efficacy but also minimizes adverse reactions, ensuring that medications work harmoniously with a patient's genetic code.

Moreover, AI facilitates the continuous refinement of genomic research and treatment protocols. As genomic databases expand, AI systems learn and adapt, constantly enhancing their predictive capabilities. This iterative learning process signifies that personalized genomics will continue to evolve, becoming increasingly precise and sophisticated. The potential to adjust treatment strategies dynamically as new information emerges is a leap forward from traditional static methodologies.

The implications of personalized genomics with AI extend into public health as well. The ability to predict and manage risks on an individual level scales up to populations, offering a chance to address and mitigate widespread health issues. With AI's predictive prowess, healthcare systems can allocate resources more efficiently, prioritize high-risk groups, and potentially curb the advance of diseases with targeted interventions.

Despite these remarkable advancements, the integration of AI in personalized genomics doesn't come without challenges. Ensuring accuracy in AI predictions and maintaining the integrity of genomic data are critical concerns. The sensitivity of genetic data necessitates stringent privacy protocols to protect individuals' information while enabling the sharing of data that fuels AI learning. This delicate balance requires rigorous ethical oversight and robust technological safeguards.

Ethical considerations also extend into the realm of accessibility. As AI-driven genomics becomes more prevalent, it's crucial to address disparities in access to these sophisticated medical innovations. Ensuring that personalized genomic insights benefit all segments of society, regardless of socioeconomic status, is vital in avoiding a deepening of healthcare inequalities.

To truly harness the transformative power of personalized genomics with AI, collaboration across disciplines is essential. It's a multi-faceted endeavor involving geneticists, bioinformaticians, AI specialists, and healthcare providers. This interdisciplinary synergy is what will drive the field forward, facilitating continuous innovation and the translation of genomic discoveries into practical health solutions.

Personalized genomics with AI may still be in its early stages, but its potential is boundless. As AI technology advances and our understanding of the genome deepens, the vision of a future where healthcare is as unique as our very DNA is no longer a distant dream. It's a burgeoning reality that's reinventing how we approach medicine, with each individual serving as both the subject and the beneficiary of these incredible developments.

Ultimately, AI in personalized genomics holds the power to not only revolutionize how we understand and treat diseases but also to redefine our very approach to health. It embodies the promise of precision medicine, where the convergence of technology and human biology meets, creating a tailored path to health that's uniquely suited to each person's genetic story. As we continue to explore and expand these capabilities, the frontier of personalized genomics will undoubtedly continue to push the boundaries of what is possible in healthcare.

Chapter 11:
Ethical Considerations
in AI Healthcare

As AI becomes an integral part of healthcare, ensuring ethical practices isn't just a responsibility—it's a necessity. The surge in AI-driven technologies has outpaced traditional ethical frameworks, prompting urgent discussions around privacy, data security, and algorithmic bias. The delicate balance between innovation and ethical considerations is not easily achieved, yet it's crucial for patient autonomy and trust. Concerns over data breaches highlight the need for robust security measures that protect sensitive health information, while biases in AI algorithms pose risks of perpetuating inequalities in healthcare outcomes. Addressing these issues requires collaboration among technologists, ethicists, and healthcare providers to develop fair, transparent, and accountable AI systems. Ultimately, forging a path forward means committing to ethical diligence as fervently as we chase technological brilliance, ensuring AI advancements benefit all individuals equitably.

Privacy Concerns and Data Security

As artificial intelligence embeds itself more deeply into the fabric of healthcare, the issues of privacy concerns and data security rise to the forefront of ethical considerations. The allure of AI and its potential to revolutionize patient care rests heavily on the access to vast amounts of sensitive data. This symbiotic relationship between technology and data makes it crucial to scrutinize how information is gathered, stored, and used. After all, in the healthcare domain, trust is as vital as treatment.

With every digital footprint left in patient records, algorithms learn and evolve. The capability of AI to offer insights and anticipate health issues before they manifest is undeniably appealing. However, a significant challenge lies in ensuring that the intimate details of a patient's health history remain confidential. A breach of data not only risks personal embarrassment but in severe cases, could also subject individuals to discrimination in employment or insurance contexts.

The multifaceted nature of AI systems necessitates leveraging various data sources, ranging from electronic health records (EHRs) and insurance claims to genomic information and social determinants of health. Each of these data streams carries its own set of privacy challenges. For instance, genomic data offers profound insights into individual predispositions to certain diseases, but is extremely sensitive. Misuse or unauthorized access could potentially influence life decisions about procreation or insurance long before these diseases manifest.

Another fundamental issue is the security infrastructure that supports AI in healthcare. As systems grow more integrated and sophisticated, the surface area exposed to potential attacks also expands. Cybersecurity measures must evolve in tandem with AI advancements. Developing robust, impenetrable security architectures is not just a reactive measure; it is foundational to maintaining patient trust in digital health solutions.

Encryption stands out as a cornerstone in the battle against unauthorized data access. By converting data into a coded format, encryption ensures that only those with the appropriate keys can decipher the stored information. Despite its efficacy, encryption alone isn't foolproof. It must be part of a broader security strategy that includes multi-factor authentication, continuous monitoring, and regular security audits to stay a step ahead of potential threats.

Moreover, ethical data handling isn't solely about protection from external threats. It also encompasses ensuring that partnerships formed between healthcare providers and AI firms are transparent and consensual. Patients should have a clear understanding of how their data will be used and must provide informed consent. Consent models need to be more dynamic than their current static forms, possibly allowing granular control over what specific parts of their data can be shared and for what purpose.

The concept of 'data minimization' is gaining traction among privacy advocates. This principle emphasizes that only the minimum necessary data should be collected and retained for AI processes. By limiting data collection, the potential fallout from a breach can be significantly reduced. However, the balance is delicate, as overly restrictive data practices can stifle the progress of AI development, leading to a gap in potentially life-saving innovations.

Furthermore, the emergence of technologies such as federated learning offers a promising pathway. By allowing AI models to be trained on decentralized data without the need to centralize patient information, federated learning minimizes risks associated with data transfer and aggregation. These technologies are a stepping stone in maintaining a balance between leveraging vast datasets and preserving individual privacy.

The implications of GDPR (General Data Protection Regulation) and similar regulations introduce an added layer of complexity and assurance. While these laws were instituted in part to protect patient rights in an increasingly digital landscape, they also come with challenges. Complying with varying global data protection regulations can prove arduous for AI-driven healthcare initiatives that operate across multiple jurisdictions. Yet, when adhered to, such regulations can set high standards for data protection, acting as beacons for ethical AI practices.

Ethics committees and institutional review boards play critical roles in overseeing the responsible implementation of AI systems in healthcare. These bodies ensure that data-related decisions are made with ethical considerations at their core. Their oversight extends to ensuring that data sharing between AI companies and healthcare entities upholds patient rights and privacy, with data anonymization and de-identification techniques being rigorously applied.

As we continue to unravel the potential of AI in healthcare, it remains imperative to acknowledge that data privacy and security are not static concerns. They demand continuous vigilance and adaptation. Engaging patients in dialogue, educating them about the impact of their data usage, and involving them in decision-making processes can fortify trust and promote a sense of partnership in their healthcare journey.

Ultimately, the journey towards integrating AI within healthcare seamlessly and ethically hinges on the industry's ability to protect the beating heart of its advancements – data. In this delicate balance of innovation and protection, lies the promise of creating a future where patients feel empowered and safeguarded, knowing their private information is handled with the utmost care and integrity.

Addressing Bias in AI Algorithms

As artificial intelligence (AI) continues to reshape healthcare, it brings along unparalleled opportunities for enhancing diagnostics, treatments, and patient care. Yet, among the myriad benefits, an underlying issue requires careful consideration: bias in AI algorithms. The presence of bias not only jeopardizes the potential of AI to deliver equitable healthcare but also raises significant ethical concerns that must be addressed to ensure that AI truly benefits all.

Bias in AI can manifest in several ways. At its core, algorithmic bias usually stems from the data used to train AI systems. If the datasets contain unbalanced or unrepresentative samples, AI models may produce skewed results that can inadvertently favor or disadvantage particular groups. For instance, if a medical AI system is trained primarily on data from one demographic, it might underperform when diagnosing conditions in patients from other backgrounds. Such discrepancies can lead to misdiagnoses, inappropriate treatments, or even detrimental patient outcomes.

Acknowledging bias in AI isn't about attributing culpability but recognizing the inherent limitations within current data structures and methodologies. Data used in training AI systems often reflect the inequalities present in the broader healthcare system. These include socioeconomic disparities, racial and gender imbalances, and historically documented biases in medical research. As a result, an AI algorithm might perpetuate existing prejudices unless specific measures are taken to identify and mitigate these biases.

Effective solutions to address bias in AI healthcare require multidimensional approaches. Firstly, data collection practices must be re-evaluated to ensure they're as inclusive and representative as possible. This involves sourcing data from diverse populations, taking into account variations in age, gender, race, socioeconomic status, and geographic location. Only through a rich diversity of data can AI systems begin to offer healthcare services that are truly equitable.

Furthermore, the implementation of bias-detection tools is vital in this journey. These tools can help identify potential biases in datasets and AI models even before they affect clinical decision-making. By thoroughly vetting the data for potential anomalies and discrepancies, healthcare providers can ensure that their AI systems function with greater fairness and accuracy. Conducting regular audits of AI systems and continuously monitoring their outcomes is another critical step in this regard.

Another promising avenue involves the development of robust algorithmic frameworks designed to 'learn' less biased pathways. Researchers are exploring innovative machine learning techniques that actively seek to minimize bias during both training and operation. Techniques such as 'fairness constraints' in model design can lead to more balanced and unbiased AI systems. These constraints require the algorithm to weigh different outcomes equally, rather than optimize for a single metric or demographic, thus fostering inclusivity in its recommendations.

Ethical oversight plays a quintessential role in mitigating bias. It's essential that governments, regulatory bodies, healthcare institutions, and the AI communities collaborate to establish guidelines and standards for ethical AI deployment. Regulatory frameworks need to be adaptive and capable of addressing the rapid advancements in AI technologies without stifling innovation. Such regulations should prioritize transparency, accountability, and equitable access, ensuring AI serves as an impartial assistant to healthcare providers.

Open-source AI initiatives can also be instrumental. By providing access to tools and algorithms, the broader AI and healthcare communities can contribute to refining and improving models collaboratively. This transparency not only fosters trust but also encourages a communal approach to identifying and rectifying biases. Open collaborations provide opportunities for cross-validation of models and enable peer reviews that bring diverse perspectives to the table.

Furthermore, involving interdisciplinary teams in the creation and oversight of AI systems is crucial. Collaborations between data scientists, clinicians, ethicists, sociologists, and patient advocacy groups can offer comprehensive insights into the various facets of AI implementation. These teams collectively ensure the alignment of technology with the cultural, ethical, and social values intrinsic to healthcare.

Patient advocacy must also take center stage in addressing AI bias. Patients have a right to understand how AI tools are used in their care and the inherent limitations and risks, including potential biases. Promoting patient awareness allows individuals to advocate for their health actively and push for the adoption of fairer AI practices across healthcare systems.

The journey towards unbiased AI in healthcare is complex and long. However, with persistent efforts in research, regulatory foresight, and community initiatives, the healthcare sector can leverage AI technologies to offer universally equitable healthcare solutions. Addressing bias isn't merely about mitigating risks; it's about honing AI as a tool that recognizes and elevates human dignity, fostering an inclusive and empathetic healthcare environment for all patients.

Ultimately, as AI becomes embedded deeply within medical practices, its success will hinge on our collective ability to use it responsibly and justly. Transparent practices, ethical diligence, and continuous dialogue among all stakeholders are pivotal in harnessing AI's transformative capabilities, ensuring its equitable application across the vast landscape of human healthcare needs.

Chapter 12:
AI in Telemedicine

The remarkable fusion of artificial intelligence and telemedicine is proving to be a game-changer in expanding healthcare access and reshaping patient experiences. This synergy isn't just about replacing in-person consultations with video calls; it's about leveraging AI to analyze data, predict patient needs, and ensure timely interventions. By integrating AI, virtual health services transcend geographical barriers, bringing quality care to underserved areas and optimizing practitioner workflows. With innovations like AI-driven chatbots, predictive analytics, and remote monitoring tools, telemedicine becomes a powerhouse for proactive health management and personalized patient interactions. These advancements pave the way for a more equitable healthcare system, where accessibility and efficiency are no longer mutually exclusive but instead work hand in hand to enhance outcomes for all.

Expanding Access to Care

Telemedicine has emerged as a pivotal solution in the healthcare industry, wielding the power of Artificial Intelligence (AI) to break down geographical and logistical barriers that once hindered access to care. The integration of AI in telemedicine is not just a technological evolution; it's a revolution that promises to democratize healthcare by bringing high-quality services to individuals regardless of their location. This advancement is particularly crucial for those residing in remote or underserved areas where healthcare resources are scarce.

Imagine a world where a patient's location no longer restricts their access to top-tier medical expertise. This concept is fast becoming a reality through the synergy of AI and telemedicine. AI-powered telemedicine platforms enable real-time analysis and interaction, capable of supporting a wide range of clinical scenarios. They empower healthcare professionals to conduct remote consultations, monitor patient health metrics, and offer timely interventions, thereby ensuring patients do not miss out on necessary care due to accessibility issues.

AI's role in expanding access to telemedicine cannot be overstated. Algorithms that process vast amounts of data at astonishing speeds allow for the creation of intuitive and efficient platforms. These systems can triage patients, prioritize cases based on urgency, and match patients with appropriate specialists, all in a fraction of the time it would take human administrators. Clinicians can focus on what they do best—providing care—while AI handles logistics and data management.

One of the most significant benefits of AI in telemedicine is its ability to personalize patient care. Through machine learning, these systems learn from each interaction, continuously refining their recommendations and interventions. For instance, AI can analyze past medical history alongside real-time data to predict potential complications, offering preemptive advice or alerts to both doctors and patients. This level of personalization enhances patient outcomes and satisfaction, turning patients into active participants in their own healthcare journey.

Moreover, AI in telemedicine facilitates continuity of care by creating a seamless interface between virtual and in-person consultations. Patients can start their treatment plans with a telehealth visit and transition to physical consultations when necessary without losing important medical history or insights captured during digital appointments. This continuity helps in building a comprehensive view of the patient's health and fosters long-term health management rather than isolated, episodic care interventions.

The rise of AI-enhanced telemedicine is especially transformative for chronic disease management. For patients managing conditions like diabetes or hypertension, regular monitoring and timely intervention are crucial. AI-driven telemedicine tools can continuously monitor vital signs and medication adherence, providing real-time alerts to healthcare providers if anomalies are detected. This proactive management can prevent complications and hospital admissions, ultimately reducing healthcare costs and improving patient quality of life.

Furthermore, the integration of AI in telemedicine promotes educational empowerment among communities with limited access to educational resources. AI systems can provide patients with tailor-made educational content that helps them better understand their conditions, treatments, and lifestyle adjustments needed to improve their health. This can significantly enhance informed decision-making capabilities, allowing patients to take charge of their healthcare with confidence.

In addition to the aforementioned benefits, AI in telemedicine also addresses the critical shortage of healthcare professionals in many regions. By facilitating virtual consultations and diagnostics, AI can alleviate the burden on overextended healthcare systems, enabling a more equitable distribution of medical expertise across various demographics. This approach ensures that even those in the most isolated areas can access care that was once considered a privilege of urban centers.

Despite these advancements, challenges remain in fully realizing the potential of AI within telemedicine. Infrastructure deficiencies, regulatory hurdles, and data security concerns need addressing to pave the way for broader adoption. However, ongoing innovations in data encryption and regulatory frameworks are continuously improving, assuring stakeholders of the path forward.

In conclusion, the expansion of care through AI-driven telemedicine heralds a new era in healthcare, one defined by inclusivity, efficiency, and precision. This transformation not only promises to improve patient outcomes but also redefines the very nature of accessibility to healthcare, making quality medical care a reality for everyone, everywhere. The compassionate application of this technology nurtures a future where health inequities can be systematically dismantled, offering hope and healing in new, impactful ways.

Innovations in Virtual Health

The landscape of telemedicine has been radically transformed by the integration of artificial intelligence (AI), unveiling a new era of virtual health innovations. As AI intertwines with healthcare, it's reshaping how medical practitioners, tech-savvy innovators, and patients perceive and engage with health services. In an age where convenience and efficiency reign supreme, AI-driven strategies are redefining patient interactions, clinical assessments, and comprehensive care delivery.

AI's influence in virtual health is multifaceted, extending from simple chatbots to complex algorithms that predict patient outcomes. Virtual consultations, powered by sophisticated AI tools, offer a glimpse into the future where geography no longer dictates access to quality healthcare. This has profound implications for those in remote or underserved areas, allowing them to tap into specialized care that was once out of reach.

Imagine a scenario where AI algorithms trawl through vast quantities of medical data in milliseconds to aid doctors during virtual consultations. This isn't a distant dream — it's happening today. AI-assisted platforms provide clinicians with real-time insights, enabling them to make informed decisions swiftly. This blend of AI's analytic prowess with human intuition enhances diagnostic accuracy and tailors treatments to individual patient needs.

With the advent of machine learning and natural language processing, virtual assistants and chatbots are becoming integral components of telemedicine. These tools engage with patients to schedule appointments, offer preliminary diagnoses, and even provide post-treatment follow-ups. This not only eases clinicians' workloads but also empowers patients to manage their health proactively.

Furthermore, AI has been instrumental in developing virtual triage systems. These systems can evaluate a patient's symptoms and medical history, offering preliminary assessments that can prioritize cases based on urgency. Such innovations cut down waiting times and steer critical care resources where they are needed most, ultimately saving lives.

One significant leap forward is the use of AI in remote patient monitoring. Wearable devices equipped with AI algorithms track vital signs and health metrics continuously, alerting healthcare providers to any anomalies in real-time. This constant monitoring isn't just about data collection; it's a dynamic process that contributes to ongoing patient management, providing peace of mind and added security.

Telemedicine platforms utilizing AI now offer predictive analytics that empower patients and doctors alike to anticipate potential health issues. By analyzing patterns and trends in patient data, AI can forecast complications before they arise, paving the way for preventive interventions. This shift from reactive to proactive care marks a pivotal transformation in healthcare approach.

AI's ability to handle large datasets efficiently also aids in the personalization of health advice. Virtual health assistants can offer personalized recommendations regarding diet, exercise, medication, and lifestyle choices, tailored to each individual's genetic makeup and health profile. This personalized approach not only improves patient outcomes but also increases patient engagement by making health advice relevant and actionable.

The evolution of AI in virtual health also brings enhanced decision-support systems for clinicians. By leveraging AI's capacities for data analysis and pattern recognition, doctors can access suggested diagnoses and treatment plans, informed by a vast repository of medical literature and patient data. These insights supplement the physician's expertise, reducing the margin for error and enhancing care quality.

However, the expanded role of AI in virtual health is not without challenges. Ensuring data privacy and security remains paramount as these systems handle sensitive patient information. Robust encryption methods and compliance with healthcare regulations such as HIPAA are necessary to maintain trust and protect patient confidentiality.

Furthermore, addressing the digital divide is critical to the widespread adoption of AI in virtual health. While technology races ahead, equitable access must be ensured, bridging gaps between different populations and regions. Investments in digital infrastructure and education will be crucial in making state-of-the-art virtual health services universally accessible.

The ethical implications of AI in telemedicine continue to prompt debates among healthcare professionals, ethicists, and technologists. Questions about algorithmic transparency, the risk of bias in AI decision-making, and the implications of machine-led diagnostics are rightly subject to scrutiny and ongoing discussion.

In summary, the innovations brought about by AI in virtual health are transformative, heralding an age where medical care is not only more efficient but also more accessible. These breakthroughs hold great promise for fundamentally altering how care is delivered, making healthcare a more equitable and patient-centered industry. As AI technologies mature, collaboration between experts from different fields will be indispensable in navigating the complexities and maximizing the benefits for all stakeholders involved in this healthcare revolution.

Chapter 13:
AI and Healthcare Administration

In the realm of healthcare administration, AI is emerging as a catalyst for transformation, streamlining operations like never before. By automating routine tasks and reducing human error, AI enables healthcare professionals to focus on what truly matters—patient care. From managing electronic health records to optimizing supply chains, AI-driven solutions are alleviating administrative burdens, allowing institutions to operate more efficiently. The integration of predictive analytics offers a proactive approach to resource allocation, ensuring that healthcare providers are better prepared to meet patient needs and improve outcomes. As AI continues to evolve, its role in healthcare administration promises a future where efficiency and precision are not just aspirational but achievable, leading to a more patient-centered healthcare ecosystem.

Streamlining Operations with AI

In the rapidly evolving landscape of healthcare, artificial intelligence (AI) has emerged as a transformative force in administrative operations. By automating and optimizing various processes, AI reduces inefficiencies and enhances productivity within healthcare facilities. From scheduling and inventory management to patient billing and beyond, AI's capabilities are vast and expanding, offering solutions that appear both innovative and practical.

One of the key areas where AI is making a significant impact is in managing patient schedules and streamlining appointments. Traditionally, scheduling involved manual input and coordination, often resulting in human error and inefficiencies. AI-driven systems now have the ability to learn patterns and preferences, optimizing schedules to reduce waiting times and balance staff workloads. These systems can predict high-demand periods, allowing administrators to allocate resources more effectively. They consider a plethora of variables—such as patient preferences, provider availability, and past no-show rates—to ensure appointment systems are both robust and patient-centric.

Inventory management in healthcare facilities is another area where AI has proven invaluable. With countless medical supplies and pharmaceuticals in constant flux, maintaining optimal stock levels can be a daunting task. AI systems now employ sophisticated algorithms to track inventory use, predict future needs, and automate reordering processes. This not only minimizes the risk of stockouts and overstocking but also frees up staff to focus on patient care rather than administrative burdens. The ripple effect of these improvements extends to reducing wastage and lowering operational costs, creating a more sustainable healthcare environment.

Financial operations in healthcare stand to gain significantly from AI's capabilities. Billing processes, often fraught with errors due to the complexity of insurance policies, coding, and regulations, can be streamlined using AI. These systems can categorize and code bills with high accuracy, ensuring that claims are processed swiftly and accurately. By automating these tasks, healthcare providers can reduce the incidence of denied claims and shorten revenue cycles, ultimately improving financial health and patient satisfaction.

The administrative workforce itself benefits from AI's integration into healthcare operations. By automating routine and repetitive tasks,

AI enables administrative staff to focus on more strategic and human-centered roles. This shift not only enhances job satisfaction but also fosters a work environment focused on innovation and empathy rather than clerical monotony. Additionally, AI can serve as a decision-support tool, providing insights and analytics that help administrators make informed decisions swiftly.

AI is also ushering in a new era of data management within healthcare administration. The sheer volume of data generated daily in healthcare is staggering, and managing this data is crucial for operational excellence. AI-driven solutions can sift through this data with unparalleled speed and precision, extracting meaningful insights that inform policy-making, strategic planning, and quality improvement initiatives. This level of data analysis enables healthcare organizations to identify trends, forecast needs, and optimize resource allocation, paving the way for data-driven decision-making.

Security is a paramount concern when it comes to healthcare data, and AI plays a vital role in safeguarding this sensitive information. Advanced AI systems enhance cybersecurity by monitoring network traffic for suspicious activity, predicting potential vulnerabilities, and providing real-time alerts to preempt data breaches. This proactive approach not only protects patient data but also ensures compliance with regulatory standards, such as HIPAA, which protect patient information.

One cannot ignore the ethical dimensions of AI in streamlining healthcare operations. Decision-makers must balance technological advancement with ethical considerations, ensuring that AI applications are equitable and transparent. For instance, algorithms used in administrative tasks should be free from bias and designed to enhance inclusivity rather than inadvertently marginalizing any group. Ongoing evaluation and auditing of AI systems are crucial to maintaining integrity and trust in their deployment.

As healthcare continues to evolve, the role of AI in streamlining operations will undoubtedly expand. Future innovations may bring even more sophisticated integrations, such as AI systems capable of real-time language translation to support diverse patient populations, enhancing communication, and accessibility. Moreover, the development of AI-driven predictive models can further improve resource allocation and emergency preparedness, anticipating needs and augmenting responsiveness.

The pathway to fully leveraging AI in healthcare administration is not without hurdles. Integrating AI into existing systems requires significant investment, both financially and in terms of time and training. Organizations must commit to not only implementing these technologies but also to cultivating a culture that embraces change and continuous learning. It is this commitment that will ultimately determine the success and sustainability of AI applications in healthcare.

Looking ahead, it is clear that AI holds the potential to revolutionize healthcare administration, transforming operations from the ground up. By automating repetitive tasks, enhancing data management, and optimizing resource allocation, AI creates a framework poised for efficiency and excellence. As stakeholders continue to innovate and collaborate, AI stands ready to unveil new horizons in the practice of modern healthcare, making systems smarter and more patient-focused than ever before. The future of healthcare administration, with AI at its core, promises a dynamic landscape where technology and human touch coexist harmoniously to serve the greater good.

Reducing Administrative Burden

In the complex ecosystem of healthcare, administrative tasks have long been a notorious burden. They demand time, resources, and energy, which can otherwise be spent on patient care. However, artificial intelligence (AI) is poised to transform this scenario significantly. It has the potential to streamline operations, optimize efficiency, and notably reduce the administrative workload that often bogs down healthcare professionals. This transformation is not just about efficiency; it's about reshaping the role of healthcare providers, allowing them more time to focus on what truly matters: patient interaction and care.

The volume of data managed in healthcare facilities is astounding. From patient records to insurance claims and scheduling, the sheer amount of paperwork is daunting. AI technologies, such as machine learning and natural language processing, can automate data entry, categorize information, and even predict future administrative needs. These tools act as administrative assistants, tirelessly working behind the scenes to ensure smooth operations without human error.

Consider the use of AI in scheduling and appointment management. Advanced algorithms analyze patterns, predict no-shows, and optimize appointment slots. This ensures that time is utilized effectively, reducing waiting periods for patients while maximizing the productivity of healthcare providers. Furthermore, AI systems can send automated reminders to patients, decreasing missed appointments and enhancing overall service accessibility. The result? A more fluid schedule that's both responsive and adaptive to real-time changes.

Billing and claims processing is another area where AI demonstrates its prowess. By automating these processes, AI significantly reduces the time and cost involved. The systems can swiftly and accurately process insurance claims, ensuring compliance with the latest regulations and minimizing the likelihood of error. This not only accelerates the revenue cycle but also minimizes the stress associated with financial processes in healthcare management.

The integration of AI into electronic health records (EHR) has been another pivotal development. AI can extract and synthesize data from EHRs, providing healthcare professionals with accessible insights at the click of a button. Automated data entry reduces the risk of incomplete or inaccurate patient records, ensuring that critical information is both comprehensive and current. With these capabilities, healthcare providers can spend less time on documentation and more time on direct patient care—a shift that leads to more meaningful interactions and improved patient satisfaction.

Moreover, AI is enhancing compliance and report generation functions. Healthcare facilities need to adhere to a complex web of regulations and standards. Here, AI simplifies the process, continuously scanning databases to ensure compliance with the latest laws and generating detailed reports with ease. This capability diminishes the administrative burden on staff, who would otherwise need to invest countless hours in regulatory compliance and reporting activities.

AI's role as an aggregator of information is also revolutionizing collaboration within healthcare systems. By providing a unified platform where different departments can seamlessly exchange information, AI fosters a collaborative environment that was previously difficult to achieve. IT systems equipped with AI capabilities can detect anomalies or discrepancies in data, quickly flag them for review, and suggest corrective action. This ensures that common administrative hurdles, such as inconsistent data entries or communication breakdowns, are swiftly and efficiently addressed.

Of course, as we embrace AI's promise, we must navigate its thoughtful integration into existing systems. Successful deployment in healthcare administration depends on meticulous planning, addressing workforce training needs, and fostering a culture that embraces technological change. This requires both investment in AI technologies and a commitment to fostering an ongoing partnership between humans and machines.

As AI continues to evolve, it holds the promise of even greater efficiencies. Future developments could see AI systems capable of more complex decision-making, offering strategic insights drawn from vast datasets to inform policy and operational improvements. This vision represents an era where administrative tasks are no longer seen as burdensome, but rather as opportunities for strategic innovation and improvement in care delivery.

While the efficiencies brought by AI are staggering, they come with significant responsibility and ethical considerations. Ensuring transparency in processes, maintaining patient privacy, and preventing algorithmic bias are critical areas that require continuous attention and innovation. Yet, the ultimate goal remains clear: to cut through administrative clutter, allowing healthcare professionals to redirect their focus from paperwork to patient care, enriching the healthcare experience for both provider and patient alike.

As AI reshapes the administrative landscape, the potential to redefine healthcare itself is enormous. By alleviating a significant portion of the administrative burden, AI empowers healthcare professionals to re-invest their skills and compassion where they are needed most—ushering in a more efficient, effective, and patient-centered era of healthcare administration.

Chapter 14:
AI in Emergency Medicine

In the high-stakes world of emergency medicine, where every second counts, artificial intelligence is proving to be a game-changer. As we continue to push the boundaries of what's possible, AI is stepping into roles that demand not just speed but also precision and adaptability. From advanced algorithms that instantly analyze patient data to identify critical conditions, to AI-driven tools that aid in triaging and managing resources during a mass casualty event, the integration of AI systems is reshaping how emergency departments respond to crises. The fusion of human expertise with AI capabilities is enabling healthcare professionals to predict patient needs more effectively, reduce wait times, and improve outcomes in life-or-death situations. Not only is AI enhancing the efficiency of emergency response, but it's also opening doors to new methods of treatment and care that were once thought unimaginable. As AI continues to evolve, its role in emergency medicine promises a future where the intersection of technology and human intervention leads to unprecedented levels of care and compassion. While challenges and ethical considerations remain, the potential benefits of AI in this field are a compelling call to action for continued innovation and collaboration.

Rapid Response and AI

In the high-stakes world of emergency medicine, every second counts. The rapid response required in critical situations often means the difference between life and death. It's in this realm that artificial intelligence (AI) is making some of the most significant impacts—and it's not just about speed. AI's involvement in emergency medicine is reshaping the landscape by offering unprecedented accuracy, efficiency, and support, helping healthcare professionals respond more effectively to crises.

Emergency departments (EDs) are often chaotic and unpredictable. Given the urgency that defines them, it's imperative that decisions are made swiftly and correctly. AI algorithms are designed to process vast amounts of data in real-time, sifting through patient records, lab results, and even ongoing vital sign monitoring. By doing so, AI systems can predict potential complications and suggest treatment plans almost instantaneously. This not only accelerates the decision-making process but also allows healthcare professionals to focus their expertise where it's needed most—direct patient care.

One important domain where AI is extending its capabilities is in triage, the process of determining the priority of patients' treatments based on the severity of their conditions. Traditional triage relies heavily on a nurse's experience and the initial information provided, which can sometimes lead to human error due to the overwhelming nature of emergency settings. AI augments this process by quickly analyzing critical variables and recommending prioritization based on real-time data and historical precedent. This ensures that patients with time-sensitive issues receive immediate attention.

Additionally, AI's role in predictive analytics has proven invaluable in emergency scenarios. For instance, systems equipped with machine learning algorithms can anticipate surges in patient arrivals based on historical data and external factors like local events or seasonal patterns. By predicting these influxes, healthcare facilities can better prepare by allocating resources, such as staff and equipment, thereby reducing wait times and improving patient outcomes. It's a vision of proactive rather than reactive healthcare management that AI is making possible.

AI's ability to integrate with wearable technology and mobile apps is another innovative advancement. These tools empower patients to take an active role in their health monitoring, providing crucial real-time data to emergency responders. Consider a scenario where a patient's wearable device detects an anomaly in heart rate or blood pressure, immediately relaying this information to the nearest ED. Emergency medical techs can prepare for the patient's arrival ahead of time, informed by AI-driven insights, potentially administering life-saving interventions sooner.

Moreover, language barriers in diverse populations can significantly impede rapid response and accurate diagnosis in emergencies. AI-driven translation tools and smart assistants equipped with natural language processing capabilities are transforming communication within EDs. They facilitate instant translations of patient symptoms and medical histories into the language of the attending healthcare provider, minimizing misunderstandings and enhancing patient care.

In the midst of the COVID-19 pandemic, AI showcased its capabilities in crisis management. AI-based predictive models were developed to distribute ventilators effectively, forecast ICUs' capacity needs, and identify high-risk patients using data patterns from electronic health records. These models guide emergency response teams to make informed decisions quickly, which helps save lives when medical resources are stretched thin.

However, integrating AI into emergency medicine also poses unique challenges. Accuracy is paramount, and while AI systems are exceedingly precise, they operate based on the data fed into them. Flawed or incomplete data can lead to incorrect predictions or recommendations. Therefore, maintaining high-quality data standards is essential. In addition, the question of accountability arises—when AI makes an error, who is responsible? As AI becomes more autonomous, this is a significant ethical and legal consideration that the medical community must address.

The cultural shift towards AI also requires thorough training for emergency medicine personnel. It's not just about understanding how to use new tools but learning to trust their recommendations. Confidence in AI systems comes from transparency and demonstrating consistent accuracy over time. Training programs that focus on the interplay between AI technology and human expertise will be critical in fostering this trust.

Despite these challenges, the opportunities AI presents in emergency medicine are transformative. It is not about replacing medical professionals but around enhancing their capabilities, empowering them to make better decisions swiftly. In turn, this leads to improved patient outcomes and saves more lives.

As AI continues to evolve and mature, its integration into emergency care will likely expand. Innovations such as autonomous drones equipped with AI algorithms hold the potential for delivering medical supplies to remote or inaccessible areas during emergencies. Similarly, AI-driven virtual reality simulations are already being used to train first responders in complex emergency scenarios, enhancing their preparedness and response capabilities.

Ultimately, the fusion of rapid response methodologies with AI technology marks a new era in medicine—one where patient outcomes are significantly improved through enhanced accuracy and efficiency. The potential for AI in emergency medicine is vast and promising, heralding a future where healthcare systems are more resilient, responsive, and capable of addressing the demands of modern medical emergencies.

Tools for Crisis Management

In the fast-paced world of emergency medicine, where every second counts, the integration of artificial intelligence (AI) has begun to transform how medical crises are managed. AI's ability to process vast amounts of data rapidly and its potential to enhance decision-making are crucial assets in scenarios where timely interventions can save lives. The emergence of AI-driven tools tailored specifically for crisis management is revolutionizing emergency medicine's strategies and capabilities.

At the forefront of this transformation are advanced predictive analytics systems that can identify potential emergency scenarios before they fully develop. These systems analyze patterns from historical data to forecast potential crises, allowing healthcare providers to allocate their resources more efficiently. For instance, by predicting the likelihood of increased emergency room visits due to seasonal illnesses or public events, hospitals can prepare in advance, ensuring that beds, staff, and medical supplies are appropriately allocated.

AI-powered triage systems represent another significant tool in crisis management. These systems prioritize patient care by rapidly analyzing symptoms and vital data to determine the urgency of cases. In high-pressure situations such as natural disasters or major accidents, this technology ensures that those in critical condition receive immediate attention, potentially reducing mortality rates. Machine learning algorithms enhance the accuracy of these systems, continuously learning from new data to improve triage decisions.

A key component of AI in crisis management is its role in facilitating communication and coordination among emergency response teams. AI-driven platforms can streamline information sharing across different agencies, enabling a unified response to crises. Such platforms provide real-time updates and analytics to support decision-making, ensuring that emergency services operate with maximum efficiency. The synchronization of efforts between paramedics, hospitals, and governmental agencies is crucial when responding to large-scale emergencies, and AI makes such coordination more seamless than ever before.

Natural language processing (NLP) technologies are also integral tools, enabling the rapid processing and understanding of spoken language in emergency calls. NLP systems can quickly extract key information from distress signals, even amidst background noise, ensuring that emergency responders receive vital information in a timely manner. These capabilities are particularly beneficial in high-pressure environments where clear communication is imperative.

Furthermore, AI has made significant strides in enhancing disaster management through real-time geographical data analysis. During natural calamities like hurricanes or floods, AI tools analyze satellite images and sensor data to assess damage and predict future threats. This information guides disaster response teams in deploying resources effectively, prioritizing areas in dire need of assistance. The speed and precision of AI analysis significantly improve the effectiveness of relief efforts.

Robotics, empowered by AI, are also playing an increasingly prominent role in emergency medicine. Drones equipped with AI can survey disaster zones, delivering critical supplies to inaccessible areas and providing first responders with vital information. These robotic systems are particularly valuable in hazardous environments where human access is challenging or dangerous, allowing for safer and more efficient rescue operations.

In addition, AI is pivotal in post-crisis evaluations, which are essential for improving future response strategies. By analyzing response data, AI systems identify strengths and weaknesses in existing emergency protocols. This process provides critical insights that shape improved policies and training programs for emergency personnel, ultimately leading to more resilient healthcare systems.

The integration of AI in crisis management isn't just about technological advancement; it's about augmenting human capabilities to better prepare for, respond to, and recover from emergencies. By leveraging AI's analytical power, healthcare providers can transform crisis response into a more proactive, rather than reactive, field. The result is a healthcare system that is not only more efficient but also more capable of delivering care in the most critical of moments.

However, the implementation of AI in crisis management does present challenges. Ensuring data privacy, maintaining algorithmic fairness, and building trust among medical professionals and the public are ongoing concerns that need to be addressed. Collaborative efforts between technologists, healthcare practitioners, and policymakers are essential to navigate these obstacles effectively.

Looking forward, the potential of AI tools in crisis management is vast. As technology continues to advance, these tools will become more sophisticated and integral to emergency medical services worldwide. The ongoing refinement and integration of AI systems will not only enhance our ability to handle current challenges but also prepare us for unforeseeable future emergencies. With every disaster tackled and every crisis averted, we're witnessing the dawn of a new era where AI's partnership with humanity is poised to redefine the limits of what's possible in emergency medicine.

Chapter 15:
AI in Rehabilitation

The realm of rehabilitation is being transformed by artificial intelligence, offering promising avenues for patient recovery. By integrating smart technologies, rehabilitation programs are becoming more personalized and adaptive, catering to individual patient needs and their unique recovery journeys. AI-powered systems can analyze vast datasets from patients' physical activities and health metrics, allowing for real-time adjustments and enhancements to therapeutic interventions. This means that, rather than a one-size-fits-all approach, therapists and patients can now rely on data-driven insights to optimize recovery processes. Furthermore, AI's predictive capabilities pave the way for anticipating potential setbacks or complications, enabling pre-emptive measures that can significantly bolster the efficacy of rehabilitation programs. This incredible fusion of technology and therapy promises not only to expedite recovery times but also to enhance overall patient outcomes, empowering individuals to regain independence and improve quality of life like never before.

Enhancing Recovery with AI Assistance

In the ever-evolving landscape of healthcare, rehabilitation stands out as an area ripe for innovation. Artificial Intelligence (AI) presents a myriad of opportunities to revolutionize the way patients recover from injuries, surgeries, and debilitating conditions. With AI, we're beginning to see a transformation in rehabilitation strategies, offering not only precision and personalization but also unparalleled motivation and support.

The core of AI's influence in rehabilitation comes from its ability to analyze vast amounts of data and derive insights that would be difficult, if not impossible, for humans to process alone. By collecting and evaluating data from previous cases, AI algorithms can predict outcomes and craft personalized recovery programs. This capability ensures that each recovery journey is tailored to the patient's unique needs, accounting for their medical history, genetic predispositions, and lifestyle factors.

A practical application of AI in rehabilitation is the development of smart rehabilitation devices. These devices, imbued with AI capabilities, can adapt exercises based on real-time monitoring of a patient's performance and progress. Imagine a robotic exoskeleton that dynamically adjusts resistance for muscle strengthening exercises, offering the right level of challenge at every training session. Such technology ensures not only efficiency in physical rehabilitation but also enhances patient safety by minimizing the risk of overexertion.

Moreover, AI's integration in virtual reality (VR) and augmented reality (AR) platforms opens new pathways for immersive rehabilitation experiences. These platforms can simulate real-world environments, enabling patients to engage in physical exercises that mimic day-to-day activities or sports, but in a controlled and safe manner. The gamification aspect introduced by AR and VR, powered by AI, can also significantly boost patients' motivation, making the often tedious process of rehabilitation interactive and enjoyable.

Tele-rehabilitation, another facet of AI-enhanced recovery, has gained traction thanks to the pandemic-induced acceleration of remote healthcare. AI-driven platforms facilitate remote monitoring of patients, enabling therapists to provide timely interventions. By using AI algorithms to analyze data collected from wearable devices, therapists can remotely adjust exercise regimens and offer feedback, ensuring the patient remains on the right path even from a distance.

Personalization doesn't end at physical recovery. AI systems are increasingly being used to address the mental and emotional aspects of rehabilitation. AI-driven chatbots and virtual companions provide emotional support and encouragement, acting as reliable adherence partners. They not only remind patients about their exercise routines and medication schedules but also engage them in conversations that can mitigate feelings of isolation and demotivation.

Real-time feedback, another strength of AI, allows patients to understand their own progress more intimately. Wearable devices equipped with AI analysis can give immediate insights into heart rate variability, movement patterns, or muscle activity, allowing patients to make adjustments on-the-fly or to consult with their therapists more effectively. This instant feedback loop not only enhances the physical aspect of rehabilitation but also encourages a more engaged and informed patient.

Prevention of future injuries is also an area where AI shines. By analyzing patterns in collected data, AI systems can predict the likelihood of re-injury or the emergence of related complications. This predictive capability enables healthcare professionals to implement proactive measures, such as recommending adjustments to training regimens or lifestyle changes, thereby enhancing long-term patient outcomes.

The collaboration between AI and rehabilitation practitioners is key to maximizing the benefits of these technologies. AI doesn't replace the empathy and expert judgment of humans but rather augments their capabilities. It provides the rigorous data analysis and pattern recognition that support therapists in making more informed decisions, offering a more comprehensive approach to rehabilitation care.

Integration challenges, of course, remain. Ensuring that AI systems are reliable and free from bias is crucial. Developing intuitive interfaces that are easily navigable by both healthcare providers and patients is equally important. The transition requires ongoing collaboration between technologists and healthcare professionals, along with continuous user feedback to refine these advanced tools.

Regulatory considerations are vital to ensuring patient safety in AI-driven rehabilitation. Establishing clear guidelines around data privacy and security, consent for data usage, and the ethical implications of AI in decision-making processes is essential. This helps garner trust from patients and providers alike, paving the way for broader acceptance of these innovations.

Nevertheless, the potential for AI to enhance rehabilitation is vast. It promises a future where recovery is not only quicker but more aligned with the individual aspirations and lifestyles of patients. As AI continues to advance, we're likely to see an even greater integration of AI systems that not only enhance physical recovery but holistically contribute to a patient's overall well-being.

Indeed, the journey through rehabilitation doesn't have to be an isolating or daunting experience. With AI's assistance, it can become a personalized pathway to regaining independence and fullness of life, making each step forward a testament to the synergy between human resilience and technological innovation.

Adaptive Technologies for Rehabilitation

Adaptive technologies in rehabilitation mark a pivotal evolution in therapeutic methods, transforming how patients regain their strength, independence, and quality of life following injury or illness. Through integrating artificial intelligence, rehabilitation is experiencing unprecedented advancements that offer new hope and possibilities for countless individuals.

At the heart of these technologies are intelligent systems designed to tailor rehabilitation procedures to individual needs, enhancing efficacy and patient satisfaction. AI-powered exoskeletons, for example, are becoming increasingly prominent in helping patients recover mobility lost due to spinal cord injuries or strokes. These devices use real-time feedback and machine learning algorithms to adapt to the user's movements, providing necessary support while encouraging natural motion patterns.

In addition to exoskeletons, AI-driven prosthetics have made leaps and bounds in recent years. Advanced sensors and algorithms enable these prosthetics to mimic natural limb movements more closely and adjust to the wearer's gait or activity levels. This adaptability isn't just about physical movement—AI can also be personalized to account for specific lifestyle requirements, thus broadening the range of activities available to the user and vastly improving their quality of life.

The utilization of virtual reality (VR)-based rehabilitation is another fascinating arena benefiting from adaptive AI technologies. VR environments supported by AI algorithms allow for tailored rehabilitation programs that offer immersive simulations to aid in physical and cognitive recovery. Such experiences can provide controlled yet varied scenarios that challenge and engage patients, making the often repetitive nature of rehabilitation exercises more dynamic and effective.

A particularly noteworthy application lies in neurorehabilitation, where AI systems assist in retraining brain function and managing neurological disorders. Technologies like brain-computer interfaces (BCIs) use sophisticated algorithms to interpret neural signals, enabling patients to control devices or applications using thought alone. This is profoundly impactful for individuals with severe mobility impairments, offering them a means to communicate or interact with their environment in ways previously deemed impossible.

AI's role in adaptive rehabilitation technology extends to functional electrical stimulation (FES) systems, which stimulate nerve activation to aid muscle recovery. These systems determine optimal stimulation patterns using AI to facilitate muscle strengthening or re-education post-injury. By continuously learning and adjusting based on user progress, AI ensures that rehabilitation is as efficient and effective as possible.

Further enhancing adaptability, sensor-based technologies with AI integration allow for continuous monitoring of patient progress. Wearable devices collect data on a myriad of parameters, from heart rate and movement to muscle activity. By analyzing this data, AI systems can predict rehabilitation outcomes and suggest modifications to treatment plans, ensuring that each patient's journey is unique and progressively advancing toward optimal results.

While the technological aspects are fascinating, the true revolution in adaptive technologies for rehabilitation lies in the personalized patient care they enable. By bringing AI into the rehabilitation domain, healthcare providers can better understand not just the physiological responses, but also the psychological aspects of recovery. This is vital in tailoring treatment plans that not only aim for physical rehabilitation but also account for mental well-being.

The integration of AI technology is, without a doubt, reshaping the landscape of rehabilitation, offering tailored solutions and intelligent guidance that were once a distant aspiration. It's not just about recovering what has been lost but enhancing the potential recovery to a future where capabilities may exceed previous norms.

In conclusion, adaptive technologies powered by AI are making rehabilitation increasingly personalized, efficient, and effective. As AI continues to evolve, so too will its applications in rehab, facilitating breakthroughs that promise brighter prospects for recovery. The patient-centric approach powered by these advancements supports holistic recovery, acknowledging the multifaceted journey each individual faces when rebuilding their lives post-injury.

Chapter 16:
AI for Infectious Disease Control

In the complex battle against infectious diseases, artificial intelligence (AI) is proving indispensable, providing us with unprecedented abilities to track and respond to outbreaks with speed and precision. AI's real-time data analysis capabilities have transformed how we monitor disease spread, offering dynamic maps and predictive models that help public health officials allocate resources efficiently. This tech-driven foresight is crucial, especially during pandemics, as AI helps to identify potential hotspots and simulate the impacts of different intervention strategies. By harnessing huge datasets and diverse information sources, AI not only enhances traditional epidemiology but also fosters innovative approaches to containment and prevention. The synergy between AI and infectious disease control paints a hopeful future where rapid response and tailored health measures mitigate the severity of outbreaks, ultimately saving lives and restoring communities to health faster than ever before.

AI Tools in Disease Tracking

Artificial intelligence (AI) is redefining the landscape of infectious disease control through its revolutionary tools in disease tracking. This advancement is not just beneficial but crucial, as it allows for rapid response and increased accuracy that weren't possible with traditional methods. The world is observing unprecedented levels of interconnectedness, which, while beneficial in many respects, also accelerates the spread of infectious diseases. This is where AI steps in, acting as a sentinel—vigilant and unerring in its detection capabilities.

AI-driven tools leverage vast amounts of data collected from diverse sources like social media, wearable technology, and global health organizations to accurately predict disease outbreaks. It's as if AI has a sixth sense, observing patterns and anomalies with a precision that transcends human capability. Consider the use of natural language processing algorithms that scan social media posts, online news, and even satellite images to discern early signs of potential outbreaks. This real-time scanning translates into prompt alerts and faster mobilization of resources, ultimately saving lives.

One of the standout features of AI in disease tracking is its ability to handle and analyze vast datasets to uncover hidden patterns. Machine learning algorithms sift through previously inconceivable amounts of data—demographic information, travel history, and even climate conditions—to generate predictive models. These models are capable of estimating the likelihood, timing, and potential impact of disease spread. Knowledge like this is not only empowering for public health officials but also instrumental in strategizing interventions and optimizing resource allocation.

What's truly inspiring is the collaborative nature of AI tools, interfacing seamlessly with various data systems worldwide. This integration facilitates a centralized approach to disease monitoring and control. For instance, international databases track pathogens in real time, allowing for global surveillance of infectious agents. With AI, the data doesn't just sit idle; it's active and dynamic, continuously evolving as new information comes in, highlighting areas of concern and suggesting real-time interventions.

Another exceptional application is the development of AI-driven diagnostic tools that are capable of identifying pathogens swiftly and efficiently. When coupled with disease tracking systems, these tools provide timely insights into the presence and spread of infections, allowing healthcare providers to make informed decisions. By scaling up diagnostic capabilities, AI ensures that while diseases may spread, they don't go unnoticed, providing an opportunity to mitigate further transmission.

AI's potential extends beyond prediction and diagnosis to actively curbing disease transmission. Tools driven by AI provide insights into effective containment strategies and offer simulations to understand potential outcomes of various interventions. This predictive capability aids in formulating actionable plans while also evaluating the success of current strategies. Using AI, healthcare systems can run countless scenarios, learning from each one without putting real lives at risk.

Robust visualization techniques powered by AI also play a pivotal role in tracking diseases. Graphs, heat maps, and dashboards make complex data more digestible, enabling stakeholders to comprehend evolving situations easily. Such visual tools bridge communication gaps between data scientists and decision-makers, ensuring information is not just available but actionable. Easy-to-understand data visualization empowers authorities to implement swift responses, reducing the lag time that often cripples response efforts in traditional setups.

Moreover, AI tools enhance precision in tracking animal health and surveillance systems, identifying emerging zoonotic threats before they leap into human populations. Considering that a significant portion of human infectious diseases originate from animals, this represents a critical area for intervention. AI-based models evaluate patterns within livestock and wildlife populations, predicting possible transitions into human interaction zones and providing crucial lead time to prevent widespread outbreaks.

As we move further into an era deeply intertwined with AI, it is essential to consider the ethical frameworks governing its application in disease tracking. While AI promises transparency and accuracy, there remains the challenge of handling sensitive data responsibly. Ensuring that AI implementations respect privacy while delivering public health benefits is a line that developers and policymakers must walk with care.

Real-time adaptation and continuous learning are the cornerstones of AI tools in disease tracking. These systems are not static; they evolve, incorporating new learnings and adapting to novel viruses and bacterium with fluency and adaptability. This capacity for evolution ensures that as pathogens develop resistance or mutate into new variants, AI systems remain effective, vigilant, and relevant.

Ultimately, the synergetic blend of AI in disease tracking is revolutionizing how we approach infectious disease control. Not only does it serve as a powerful tool for health professionals and policymakers, but it also acts as a beacon of hope for communities worldwide. By enabling precise, timely, and informed responses to disease outbreaks, AI is creating a future where healthcare systems are not just reactive but strategically preemptive, preventing rather than merely containing outbreaks. As these tools become more sophisticated, integrated, and ubiquitous, their capacity to transform the global public health landscape will only intensify, charting the course for safer, healthier societies.

AI Contributions in Pandemic Response

In the realm of infectious disease control, few events have underscored the importance of speed and precision in data analysis quite like a pandemic. The recent global health crises have illuminated the invaluable role artificial intelligence (AI) plays in enhancing pandemic response efforts. AI's capacity to swiftly analyze vast data sets and generate insights has revolutionized how public health authorities prepare for and respond to pandemics.

One of the key contributions of AI in pandemic response is its ability to predict outbreaks. By analyzing vast amounts of historical and current data, ranging from clinical trial outcomes to social media posts, AI algorithms can detect patterns and identify areas at risk of an outbreak. This predictive power allows for proactive measures, enabling authorities to implement targeted interventions before a crisis spirals out of control. During the COVID-19 pandemic, AI models played a crucial role in predicting the virus spread, which significantly informed public health decisions and containment strategies.

Beyond prediction, AI has been pivotal in monitoring the real-time evolution of pandemics. With its robust data processing prowess, AI helps in discerning meaningful trends from the noise, offering actionable insights into how a disease is spreading and evolving. AI's role in this capacity extends to genomic surveillance, where it aids researchers in understanding how viruses mutate over time, thereby informing vaccine development and therapeutic strategies.

Contact tracing, a fundamental aspect of controlling infectious diseases, has also been revolutionized by AI. Traditional contact tracing methods often rely on manual efforts, which can be slow and prone to errors. AI, however, can leverage mobile data and other digital footprints to efficiently identify potential contacts of infected individuals. This automated approach not only accelerates the process but also enhances its accuracy, providing public health officials with a powerful tool to contain the spread of disease.

In terms of resource allocation, AI models contribute significantly by optimizing the distribution of medical supplies and personnel. During crises, hospitals and clinics often face shortages of critical resources. AI can analyze patient data and predict demand surges, allowing hospitals to allocate resources where they are most needed. This predictive capability aids in ensuring that patients receive timely care, which is pivotal in saving lives.

Furthermore, AI-powered tools have improved the accuracy of diagnostic processes during pandemics. Rapid and precise testing is crucial in managing infectious diseases; AI algorithms have proven to enhance the sensitivity and specificity of diagnostic tests. By analyzing complex datasets from various diagnostic platforms, these tools can reduce the number of false positives and negatives, ensuring that more accurate test results are available and that appropriate measures are taken promptly.

AI's contributions also encompass enhancing communication strategies during pandemics. By processing and analyzing public sentiment through digital platforms, AI can help health communicators identify misinformation trends and develop strategies to address them swiftly. This function is vital as misinformation can spread as rapidly as a virus, undermining efforts to control an outbreak. Thus, AI not only supports public health messaging but also ensures that populations remain informed with accurate information.

Moreover, AI has redefined the landscape of vaccine research and development. Traditionally, the process of creating vaccines has been laborious and time-consuming. However, AI algorithms accelerate this process by simulating interactions between viral proteins and potential drugs, thereby identifying promising vaccine candidates more rapidly. This capability was notably demonstrated during the COVID-19 pandemic, where AI-driven insights contributed to the unprecedented speed of vaccine development.

The ethical considerations surrounding the use of AI in pandemic response are also significant. While AI's capabilities offer incredible potential, they must be harnessed with caution to protect individual privacy. The indiscriminate collection and use of personal data can infringe upon privacy rights, creating ethical dilemmas. Therefore, striking a balance between leveraging AI and upholding ethical standards remains imperative.

The use of AI in pandemics has sparked a global dialogue on the need for collaborative frameworks and data-sharing agreements. AI's effectiveness depends largely on the quality and breadth of data available. Thus, international cooperation beyond geopolitical boundaries is necessary to ensure that data access and sharing facilitate the global monitoring of infectious diseases, enhancing collective pandemic responsiveness.

As we have seen, AI has dramatically enhanced pandemic response capabilities, offering tools that are faster and more precise than traditional methodologies. From predicting outbreaks to accelerating vaccine development, AI's contributions are diverse and profound. The evolution of AI technologies will continue to improve our readiness and response to future pandemics, marking a new era in public health where digital intelligence plays a central role in protecting human health.

AI's integration into pandemic response strategies exemplifies how advanced technologies can revolutionize public health practices. Realizing the full potential of AI in this context requires ongoing investment in AI research and infrastructure, as well as a commitment to addressing ethical concerns and fostering global cooperation. As we move forward, these investments will be essential to ensuring that AI serves as a force for good in the continuous battle against infectious diseases.

Chapter 17:
AI in Medical Education

In the dynamic realm of medical education, AI is carving new pathways for teaching and learning, reshaping how future healthcare professionals approach their studies. By integrating AI tools into curricula, students gain access to personalized learning experiences and data-driven insights that foster deeper understanding. Interactive platforms, powered by AI, simulate real-world scenarios, allowing learners to hone diagnostic and decision-making skills in a safe, virtual environment. These technological advancements not only enhance comprehension and retention but also prepare students for the complexities of modern medicine. The future of medical education promises a seamless blend of traditional methods and AI-driven innovations, equipping the next generation with a profound blend of knowledge and technological proficiency that will be pivotal in transforming patient care delivery worldwide.

Training the Next Generation with AI

As artificial intelligence increasingly finds its place in medical practice, it's imperative that we focus on training the next generation of healthcare professionals to work alongside these advanced technologies. AI in medical education not only equips students with cutting-edge skills but also fosters a new era of medical practitioners who are as adept in coding and data interpretation as they are in bedside manners. The future of medicine demands professionals who can seamlessly integrate AI into patient care, making training essential for current and future students in the medical field.

In medical schools worldwide, the curriculum is evolving to incorporate AI principles and applications. Gone are the days when medical education was solely about anatomy, pathology, or pharmaceuticals. Now, the curriculums are being expanded to include modules on data science, machine learning, and their applications in healthcare settings. This integration ensures that students not only understand the potential of AI but also see firsthand how it can revolutionize diagnostics, prognostics, and treatment strategies.

One of the most significant advantages of integrating AI into medical education is the ability to simulate real-life scenarios with unprecedented accuracy. AI-driven simulation platforms allow students to experiment with a wide range of clinical situations without the constraints of a traditional classroom or hospital setting. These simulations can provide real-time feedback and adapt to the unique learning pace of each student, creating a highly personalized education experience.

Such platforms are also vital in honing decision-making skills. Medical decisions often involve complex layers of information and the risk of human error. By training with AI-powered tools, students learn to synthesize large datasets and predict outcomes more accurately. This ability isn't taught through textbooks; rather, it's gained through experiential learning that mimics the fluidity and uncertainty of real-world patient care.

Moreover, AI serves as a bridge that spans the gap between theory and practice. It enables students to directly see the applications of theoretical knowledge in dynamic, patient-centered scenarios. For instance, while learning about cardiovascular diseases, a student could use AI algorithms to model how different treatment plans might affect patient recovery times or outcomes. The immediacy and relevance of this kind of insight are invaluable for medical students and future practitioners.

In addition to enhancing clinical skills, AI education in medicine encourages a mindset shift among future healthcare providers. It promotes a culture of continuous learning and adaptation, essential traits in a field that's as rapidly changing as healthcare. Students become accustomed to working with digital tools and data analytics, preparing them to constantly evolve and improve their practice as AI technology advances.

The importance of interdisciplinary collaboration cannot be overstated in the context of AI in medical education. Training programs are increasingly adopting a multidisciplinary approach, encouraging students to engage with experts from fields such as bioinformatics, computer science, and engineering. This exposure helps them appreciate the interconnected nature of modern healthcare solutions and prepares them to contribute innovative ideas and approaches that transcend traditional medical boundaries.

Furthermore, addressing ethical considerations will be pivotal in training the next generation. Students must be equipped not only with the technical skills to work with AI but also with a strong ethical foundation to navigate the potential dilemmas that arise from its use. This includes understanding issues related to patient privacy, the potential for bias in AI algorithms, and the importance of maintaining human oversight in decision-making processes.

Incorporating AI into medical education will also necessitate an evolution of the role of educators and mentors. Instructors will need to adapt to facilitate a learning environment where AI is a tool for exploration rather than competition. They must guide students in questioning and critically thinking about the results generated by AI, fostering an educational culture where technology augments human judgment, rather than replacing it.

The transformation of medical education through AI is not without challenges. Resource disparities between institutions can create uneven access to advanced training tools, which underscores the importance of collaboration and sharing of educational resources across institutions. Partnerships with technology companies and investments in digital infrastructure are crucial to ensuring all students can benefit from AI-integrated learning environments.

As we envision the future of healthcare, it's clear that AI-trained professionals will be at the forefront of transformative advances. These individuals will lead the charge in developing new treatments, improving patient outcomes, and expanding access to care. Training the next generation with AI empowers them with the skills, knowledge, and ethical grounding necessary to harness technology's potential while maintaining the human touch that remains at the heart of medicine.

Interactive Learning Platforms

As the integration of artificial intelligence (AI) continues to reshape medical education, one of the most transformative elements has emerged from the development of interactive learning platforms. These platforms are not just about presenting information—they bring information to life, offering an immersive experience that traditional teaching methods can't replicate.

Imagine a virtual classroom where medical students interact with AI-powered avatars simulating real patients. These avatars can express an array of symptoms, respond to various treatments, and even adapt based on the student's decisions. This type of learning doesn't merely present facts; it fosters critical thinking, decision-making, and problem-solving skills, essential for future healthcare professionals.

Interactive platforms supported by AI have revolutionized the accessibility and customization of medical training. No longer constrained by geographical boundaries, students from around the globe can access the same high-quality educational resources. These platforms adjust to the pace and learning style of each individual, providing a tailored educational experience. If a student struggles with a specific concept, the AI can identify this and provide additional resources or suggest different methods of explanation, thereby personalizing the learning journey.

The power of interactive AI platforms extends beyond the simulation of patient interactions. They incorporate diverse elements such as virtual reality (VR) and augmented reality (AR) to create dynamic and engaging content. In the setting of a virtual operating theater, for example, students can practice complex surgical techniques without the pressure and risk of a real-life scenario. The sensory involvement of VR and AR ensures that learners are not passive recipients but active participants, thereby improving retention and comprehension.

Furthermore, these interactive tools offer real-time feedback and assessment. By evaluating a student's performance against clinical standards, the AI system can pinpoint errors and offer constructive feedback instantly. This kind of immediate evaluation encourages students to learn from their mistakes and adapt their methods in subsequent simulations, promoting a deeper understanding of their future roles as healthcare providers.

The collaborative potential of AI-driven platforms also cannot be underestimated. In the medical field, teamwork is crucial, and these platforms facilitate collaborative learning through integrated social tools. Students can form study groups, discuss case studies, and even role-play as members of a healthcare team comprising various specialties. This interaction builds communication skills and the ability to work cross-functionally—an essential aspect of modern medical practice.

Moreover, AI assists educators by tracking student progress over time. With advanced analytics, instructors can identify trends and patterns in learning behaviors, allowing for adjusted curricula that meet the evolving needs of the learner. This data-driven approach not only personalizes education but also enhances the overall quality of the teaching provided.

It's also important to note the role of AI in democratizing medical education through these platforms. Students from underprivileged backgrounds or those in remote locations often face barriers in accessing quality medical training. However, AI is leveling the playing field by providing equal opportunities for learning, fostering diversity and inclusion in the medical community.

As institutions continue to adopt these platforms, we witness the emergence of a collaborative ecosystem where educators, technologists, and healthcare professionals work together to push the boundaries of medical education. This whole-system approach ensures that the development of interactive learning platforms remains aligned with the ever-evolving demands of healthcare.

Though AI-driven interactive platforms represent a significant leap forward, they also pose challenges. The initial setup of such sophisticated systems can be resource-intensive, and there's a constant need to update content to keep it aligned with the latest medical guidelines and research. Additionally, the integration of such platforms into existing curricula calls for a paradigm shift in teaching methodologies, which some institutions may find difficult to adopt.

Despite these challenges, the advantages of interactive learning platforms powered by AI outweigh the barriers. They ensure that students are not only well-versed in medical theory but also prepared for real-world application. By simulating real-life medical environments and patient interactions with an unparalleled level of realism, these platforms are setting a new standard in medical education.

In conclusion, as medical education continues to evolve, AI-powered interactive learning platforms stand at the frontier of this change. They are not only teaching tools but catalysts for redefining how we perceive and engage with medical training. As these technologies develop, the future healthcare workforce will be better equipped—armed with an education that is holistic, experiential, and profoundly impactful.

Chapter 18:
AI in Global Health Initiatives

Across continents, AI is sparking a transformation in global health initiatives, offering a beacon of hope in addressing the disparities that have long plagued healthcare. Countries from every corner of the globe are now leveraging AI to bridge gaps in medical access and optimize patient care in under-resourced regions. This innovative approach isn't just about integrating advanced technology—it's about fostering collaborations among international organizations, governments, and local communities to propel health outcomes to unprecedented heights. Both big data and machine learning play crucial roles, as these technologies analyze vast datasets to efficiently allocate resources where they're needed most, predict disease outbreaks, and tailor interventions to community-specific challenges. The ongoing partnerships and projects, while diverse in scope, all underscore a shared commitment: utilizing AI to ensure equitable healthcare access, thereby empowering even the most remote populations. Through these initiatives, AI becomes more than a tool; it evolves into a catalyst for systemic change and a pioneer of global health equity.

Bridging Gaps in Global Medical Access

In the vast landscape of healthcare, disparities in access and quality are glaringly evident. The gap between those who have timely, effective medical care and those who don't is a challenge that many regions face today. Enter artificial intelligence, a transformative ally in bridging these gaps. AI's potential to address global disparities in healthcare access isn't just theoretical; it's already being realized in practical, impactful ways.

One of AI's most promising applications in global health is its ability to break down geographical barriers. In many remote and underserved areas, access to skilled healthcare professionals is limited. AI-powered diagnostic tools can step in, offering preliminary assessments that guide patient care even when human doctors aren't immediately available. From interpreting X-rays to diagnosing skin conditions, AI algorithms are becoming valuable first-line resources.

By leveraging mobile technology, artificial intelligence is bringing healthcare solutions directly to patients' hands, literally. Smartphone applications equipped with AI can perform tasks ranging from tracking patient symptoms to recommending courses of action. For instance, maternal health apps monitoring pregnancy progress can be crucial helpers in areas with high maternal mortality rates. This isn't just about technology providing information; it's about providing life-saving guidance tailored to specific needs and contexts.

Efforts to utilize AI in optimizing supply chains for medical supplies are also crucial in closing access gaps. In resource-limited settings, the distribution of medical resources like vaccines, medications, and equipment often faces logistical hurdles. AI can dynamically predict and manage supply chain requirements, ensuring that essential resources reach the most remote corners of the world efficiently. The timely delivery of these supplies can be the difference between managing a health crisis and an unnecessary loss of life.

Telemedicine, powered by AI, is another significant leap toward universally accessible healthcare. With AI handling preliminary patient interactions, such as symptom checks and medical history analysis, healthcare providers can focus on delivering high-quality, patient-centered care. These virtual consultations enable individuals in underserved areas to connect with specialists miles away, ensuring that medical advice is not limited by distance.

Nonetheless, while AI holds great promise for bridging gaps in global medical access, deployment isn't without challenges. Internet connectivity, the backbone of most AI solutions, remains inconsistent across many regions, posing a barrier to effective implementation. Efforts to improve infrastructure must go hand-in-hand with technological deployment to maximize impact.

The implementation of AI tools must also consider cultural and linguistic contexts to ensure that technology solutions are accessible and usable by local populations. Collaborative efforts with local communities in designing AI-based healthcare solutions pave the way for tailored applications that meet specific cultural needs. Language processing technologies can help bridge communication gaps, making it easier for non-native speakers to interact with AI tools in their languages.

Furthermore, AI's role doesn't stop at diagnosis and treatment. Prognostic models powered by advanced algorithms have the capability to predict disease outbreaks, allowing quicker intervention and control. By analyzing vast datasets from various regions, AI can identify emerging patterns indicative of potential health crises. This proactive approach is particularly valuable in regions prone to endemic diseases; it allows for timely allocation of resources and preventative measures.

AI can also foster stronger global collaborations. By providing a platform to share and analyze health data transparently across borders, global researchers and healthcare providers can collectively address prevalent health issues. This collaborative spirit is crucial for tackling complex public health challenges that no single entity can solve alone.

Significantly, the ethical deployment of AI in low-resource settings must be prioritized to ensure that solutions empower rather than exploit vulnerable populations. Addressing concerns regarding data privacy and algorithmic bias is a critical step in maintaining public trust and ensuring the responsible use of AI. Here's where partnership with local organizations and ethical oversight can play pivotal roles.

Ultimately, the integration of AI into global health initiatives is a continuous journey of learning and adaptation. It requires persistent dedication to understanding the unique needs of diverse populations and developing adaptive technologies that grow along with these requirements. With AI's continued evolution, there's an opportunity to make equitable healthcare a reality for millions worldwide who currently lack it. The progress made thus far is encouraging, yet it only scratches the surface of what's possible as AI technology becomes more sophisticated and accessible over time.

As AI continues its transformative march, it holds the promise of a future where healthcare is not limited by borders or socioeconomic barriers. Bridging the gaps in global medical access isn't merely a technological endeavor; it's a humanitarian mission seeking to ensure every individual, regardless of their location or background, has the opportunity to lead a healthy, fulfilling life. As developments unfold, staying committed to the principles of equity, accessibility, and collaboration ensures that AI reaches its full potential in reshaping global health for the betterment of all.

Collaborations in AI Health Projects

As artificial intelligence continues to transform the healthcare landscape, collaborations in AI health projects stand out as a cornerstone of global efforts to improve medical access and outcomes. These partnerships bridge diverse expertise, merging cutting-edge technology with profound medical knowledge to tackle some of the world's most pressing health challenges. The convergence of AI technologies with global health initiatives paves the way for not just innovative solutions, but sustainable improvements in the public health sector.

In many ways, collaborations act as catalysts for innovation, sparking ideas that solitary efforts might not achieve. Universities, tech companies, and healthcare organizations are coming together to pool resources and knowledge. This synergy has led to the creation of AI-driven tools capable of diagnosing diseases, predicting health trends, and improving treatment personalization. One illustrative example is the collaboration between IBM and leading oncologists to harness the power of AI in cancer treatment. By analyzing vast amounts of medical literature and patient data, AI can suggest treatment plans tailored to individual patients, significantly enhancing outcomes.

The global nature of many health challenges requires a collective response. International organizations, such as the World Health Organization (WHO), have recognized the importance of collaborative AI projects in achieving health equity. Through partnerships with nations and private sectors, WHO facilitates data sharing and the development of AI tools that can address healthcare disparities. For instance, AI models that predict outbreaks of infectious diseases help deploy resources efficiently, thereby preventing epidemics from escalating.

Some of the most successful AI health collaborations involve public-private partnerships (PPPs). These alliances leverage the strengths of both sectors, balancing public interest with innovation-driven private enterprise. The Gates Foundation, for instance, has invested significantly in AI for global health projects, partnering with tech companies to develop AI solutions for malaria diagnosis and treatment. By focusing on resource-limited settings, these collaborations aim to make healthcare accessible and affordable across different demographics.

Moreover, academic institutions play a pivotal role in AI collaborations. Research universities provide a fertile ground for theoretical and practical advancements, fostering environments where AI applications can be rigorously tested and refined. Academic partnerships with tech companies and healthcare providers contribute to groundbreaking projects. Stanford University, for instance, collaborates with tech leaders to innovate in AI-driven healthcare research, pushing the boundaries of what AI can achieve in both disease detection and treatment optimization.

Yet, these collaborations face hurdles. Data interoperability and sharing constraints pose significant challenges. The integration of AI systems across different platforms and regions requires standardization and robust cybersecurity measures. Projects must navigate these complexities to ensure data can be shared safely and effectively. Addressing these issues demands policy frameworks that promote collaboration while safeguarding patient privacy and data security—an ongoing dialogue in the realm of AI health projects.

The ethical landscape is another multifaceted area requiring careful consideration. Collaborative projects need clear ethical guidelines to address issues like fairness and transparency. The involvement of diverse stakeholders in developing these guidelines is crucial, ensuring that AI tools are devoid of bias and serve all populations equitably. Transparency in AI decision-making processes remains a priority, fostering trust and acceptance amongst users worldwide.

While challenges exist, the potential benefits of collaborations in AI health projects are vast. AI-driven telemedicine initiatives, for example, are expanding access to care in rural and underserved regions by connecting patients with specialists anywhere in the world. These initiatives often depend on international collaborations to deploy technological infrastructure and train healthcare workers to utilize AI tools effectively. These efforts are especially important in low-resource settings, where AI can dramatically improve patient care quality and efficiency.

Looking ahead, it's clear that AI collaborations offer exciting possibilities for advancing global health initiatives. By fostering partnerships across borders and sectors, we can accelerate the development of solutions tailored to diverse health environments, bringing us closer to a world where quality healthcare is within everyone's reach. Such collaborations not only advance medical knowledge but also create frameworks for future innovations, embedding AI more deeply into the fabric of global health infrastructure.

In conclusion, collaborations in AI health projects exemplify the power of working together toward a common goal. They harness the strengths of disparate entities, creating a synergy that has the potential to revolutionize global healthcare as we know it. By overcoming current challenges and prioritizing ethical considerations, these collaborative endeavors can drive sustainable advancements, ensuring that the promise of AI in healthcare is realized for all.

Chapter 19:
AI in Personalized Health

In the dynamic realm of personalized health, AI shines as an unprecedented ally, transforming the way healthcare is tailored at an individual level. The integration of AI with personalized health strategies is not just about collecting data—it's about translating myriad data points into actionable, personalized insights that empower both patients and their healthcare providers. With AI-driven analytics, treatments become more precise, rehabilitation plans are finely tuned to an individual's unique health profile, and predictive algorithms identify potential health issues before they become critical. These innovations mark a shift from a one-size-fits-all approach to healthcare, spotlighting the potential of AI to revolutionize patient outcomes. As AI continues to learn and evolve, it holds the promise of crafting health solutions that are as unique as the individuals they serve, fostering a future where personalized care is the norm, not the exception.

Tailoring Health Plans with AI Insights

In today's rapidly evolving healthcare landscape, the concept of personalized health is more tangible than ever, thanks to the groundbreaking advances in artificial intelligence. AI's potential to revolutionize the way health plans are tailored is immense, offering us insights that were previously unimaginable. By diving deep into data, AI not only observes but also learns and predicts, thus enabling healthcare providers to craft health plans that are as unique as individual fingerprints.

This transformation begins with the vast amount of data that AI is able to process and analyze. Historically, health data was trapped in silos—difficult to navigate and extract meaningful insights from. Today, AI systems can integrate diverse datasets, ranging from electronic health records to genomic information, and even activity levels tracked by wearable devices. By correlating data points from different sources, AI can uncover patterns and trends that inform the customization of health plans.

Consider the example of a patient with a chronic condition, such as diabetes. Traditional health plans might focus on general management strategies and periodic check-ups. However, using AI, the plan can be meticulously tailored to predict fluctuations in blood glucose levels, suggest dietary changes, and even predict potential complications before they arise. Utilizing machine learning algorithms, AI can analyze data from continuous glucose monitors, dietary logs, and exercise patterns to offer real-time feedback and personalized health recommendations.

Moreover, AI's ability to predict health outcomes plays a critical role in creating these tailored health plans. With predictive analytics, algorithms can anticipate potential health crises based on historical data and current health metrics. For instance, AI can analyze heart rate variability, blood pressure, and patient-reported symptoms to predict the likelihood of a cardiac event. This proactive approach allows healthcare providers to implement preventive measures, which can significantly improve patient outcomes and reduce healthcare costs.

Yet, the journey of tailoring health plans with AI insights is not without its challenges. One significant hurdle is ensuring the accuracy of AI predictions. AI systems must be trained on diverse and representative datasets to minimize biases that can lead to erroneous conclusions. This requires ongoing collaboration between AI developers and healthcare professionals to refine algorithms and validate AI-generated insights through clinical trials and real-world applications.

Furthermore, the ethical implications of using AI in personalized health must be considered. Privacy concerns are at the forefront, as the data used to tailor health plans often include sensitive personal information. Ensuring robust data protection measures, securing patient consent, and clearly communicating how data is used are essential steps in building trust in AI-driven health solutions.

Interdisciplinary collaboration is key to maximizing AI's potential in personalizing health plans. By bringing together experts in medicine, data science, and technology, comprehensive strategies can be developed to harness AI's capabilities. These collaborations often lead to the creation of platforms that integrate various streams of data, creating a holistic view of a patient's health journey. Such platforms not only provide insights for healthcare providers but can also be accessed by patients to take an active role in managing their health.

Education also plays a crucial role in the successful implementation of AI-tailored health plans. Healthcare professionals must be trained to understand and interpret AI insights, ensuring that they can effectively integrate these insights into patient care. Additionally, patient education is vital to help individuals understand and trust the recommendations generated by AI systems. Empowering patients with knowledge about how AI works and how to benefit from these tools is fundamental to achieving better health outcomes.

The benefits of AI in tailoring health plans extend beyond individual care, influencing broader public health strategies. By aggregating anonymized data, AI systems can identify population health trends, helping public health officials to craft population-focused interventions and policies. For example, AI can analyze de-identified data from wearable devices to discern patterns in physical activity and nutrition, guiding public health campaigns aimed at reducing obesity and related conditions.

In conclusion, the integration of AI into the tailoring of health plans signifies a paradigm shift in modern medicine. By leveraging the power of AI insights, healthcare becomes more responsive, personalized, and preventive. As technology continues to advance, the potential for AI to transform health plans will only grow, paving the way for a future where healthcare is tailored to meet the unique needs of each individual. Through careful management of ethical concerns, continuous collaboration, and patient empowerment, we can harness the full potential of AI to improve health and well-being across diverse populations.

Predictive Analytics for Individualized Care

In the ever-evolving landscape of healthcare, predictive analytics is carving out a transformative niche, especially when it comes to individualized patient care. Through the lens of artificial intelligence (AI), predictive analytics is opening doors to deeply personalized health strategies that were once the dreams of futuristic medicine. The capacity of AI to analyze vast datasets and uncover patterns that are invisible to the human eye is setting the stage for a new era of precision health.

Predictive analytics refers to the use of data, statistical algorithms, and machine learning techniques to identify the likelihood of future outcomes based on historical data. In the context of healthcare, it means harnessing this power to predict disease risks, tailor interventions, and ultimately, improve patient outcomes. This isn't just about leveraging big data. It's about understanding individual characteristics and providing predictive insights that cater to personal health needs.

Imagine a world where your health plan is as unique as your fingerprint. This is where AI-driven predictive analytics comes into play. By sifting through oceans of patient data, from electronic health records to genomic sequences, AI creates a comprehensive profile for each individual. This means not just tracking current health conditions but predicting future health challenges. For instance, early warnings on the likelihood of developing diabetes or heart issues can spur proactive lifestyle or medical interventions.

One of the key advantages of predictive analytics is its ability to move care from reactive to proactive. Instead of waiting for symptoms to manifest, healthcare providers can anticipate and mitigate potential health issues before they become critical. This shift holds tremendous potential to alleviate strain on healthcare systems while offering patients a chance to engage in their health journey actively.

However, for predictive analytics to truly revolutionize individualized care, integration is vital. It requires a seamless merging of technology with clinical practice. AI-driven systems must be accessible and comprehensible to clinicians so that they can easily interpret and act upon the insights provided. The emphasis should be on creating tools that fit naturally within existing workflows, enhancing rather than complicating clinical decision-making.

Data privacy and security remain top priorities as well. While the benefits of predictive analytics are considerable, it also asks healthcare providers to manage sensitive patient information with the utmost care. New frameworks and regulations need to be put in place to ensure data is collected, stored, and accessed appropriately, safeguarding patients' privacy without stifling innovation.

The human element in healthcare cannot be overlooked. AI's role in predictive analytics should complement the empathetic and intuitive aspects of patient care. Although AI may offer a roadmap to potential health outcomes, the healthcare provider's role in interpreting this data and discussing it with patients is crucial. Trust between patient and provider can be strengthened when technology is used to demonstrate thoughtful and personalized care planning.

Collaboration across disciplines marks another frontier in the advancement of predictive analytics. By bringing together specialists across AI, clinical research, molecular biology, and beyond, a more holistic and robust predictive model can be created. This multidisciplinary approach is necessary to tackle the complex nature of disease and health management effectively.

AI-powered predictive analytics also holds promise beyond chronic disease management. It's revolutionizing the treatment of mental health disorders, predicting episodes of depression or anxiety, thus enabling timely interventions. In oncology, it can forecast cancer progression, aiding in choosing the most effective treatment pathways for patients. Every day, researchers are exploring new applications for these technologies, widening the scope of what personalized care can achieve.

The full realization of predictive analytics in personalized healthcare depends significantly on health information technology (HIT) infrastructure. As AI algorithms continue to grow in sophistication, the underlying HIT systems must be robust enough to support them. This may mean investing in new technologies and revamping legacy systems to build a more interconnected and agile digital health ecosystem.

Educational initiatives are equally important. As AI and predictive analytics become integral to healthcare, ongoing training for health professionals will be necessary to keep them updated on the latest advancements. This not only improves the implementation and adoption of such technologies but also ensures that the healthcare workforce remains adept at optimizing patient care.

In conclusion, predictive analytics stands at the forefront of a personalized health revolution, empowered by AI's unparalleled ability to digest and decipher complex data. The goal is not only to personalize care but also to engage patients, empower healthcare providers, and enhance healthcare systems. While challenges remain—particularly around technology integration, privacy, and education—the potential is boundless. As predictive analytics continues to evolve, it promises to shape a future where healthcare is not just personalized but profoundly proactive, with AI acting as a trusted partner in this transformative journey.

Chapter 20:
Challenges in Implementing
AI in Medicine

Navigating the integration of artificial intelligence into the intricate world of medicine poses multifaceted challenges that extend beyond mere technological hurdles. As revolutionary as AI's potential appears, the road to its full implementation is strewn with obstacles ranging from technical complexity to regulatory labyrinths. Technologies need seamless interoperability within existing systems, yet many healthcare infrastructures are fragmented and outdated, complicating AI adoption. On the regulatory front, healthcare regulators are tasked with keeping pace with rapid technological advancements while ensuring patient safety and data privacy — often an arduous and balancing act. Additionally, there's a pressing need to cultivate trust among healthcare professionals, who may be wary of relying heavily on algorithms over human judgment, and patients, who must be assured of data confidentiality and accuracy of AI-driven insights. Successfully overcoming these challenges requires a collaborative synergy among technologists, healthcare providers, policymakers, and ethicists, each contributing to a resilient framework capable of integrating AI as both a tool for innovation and a partner in care.

Overcoming Technological Barriers

The integration of artificial intelligence in medicine holds transformative potential, yet we face significant technological barriers that must be surmounted to realize its full promise. The complexity of medical data, the need for high computational power, and the challenge of integrating AI systems with existing medical technology represent formidable hurdles. Addressing these barriers requires not just cutting-edge technology, but also a strategic approach to innovation and implementation.

One of the primary challenges in implementing AI in medicine is the massive volume and complexity of data involved. The data generated from electronic health records, medical imaging, genomics, and personalized health sensors is colossal and growing exponentially. This influx of diverse, high-quality data provides an opportunity for AI systems to uncover insights previously unseen, but it also demands advanced data processing and storage solutions. Traditional databases and IT infrastructures often struggle under such burdens, necessitating technological adaptations to manage and interpret data efficiently.

AI systems rely heavily on powerful computation to perform complex algorithms needed for tasks like image recognition in radiology or predicting disease outbreaks. However, healthcare settings frequently lack the infrastructure required to support these high-performance computational demands. Implementing AI therefore involves substantial investment in computational resources and state-of-the-art technology, which can be prohibitive for many healthcare institutions. Approaches like cloud computing and distributed computing systems promise to alleviate some of these constraints by providing scalable and flexible solutions.

Integration with legacy healthcare systems presents another significant technological barrier. Hospitals and clinics often use a range of systems that vary in age, design, and function, making the integration of new AI technologies a challenging endeavor. Seamless integration is crucial to both the efficacy of AI and the safety of patients, as it must support interoperability among diverse systems while ensuring the accuracy and privacy of the data being shared. Developers and healthcare providers must work together to devise integration strategies that facilitate smooth transitions and augment existing processes without disruption.

Additionally, developing AI algorithms that are transparent, unbiased, and interpretable is crucial to overcoming technological barriers. Machine learning models often function as "black boxes," providing outcomes without clear or interpretable rationale, which can be unsuitable for medical applications. Clinicians need to understand and trust AI suggestions to incorporate them into their practice effectively. Researchers and technologists are actively working on creating models that can explain their reasoning processes and output, thereby providing clearer, more transparent decision-making pathways for healthcare professionals.

To mitigate these issues, a collaborative approach is vital. Collaboration across interdisciplinary teams, including computer scientists, healthcare practitioners, data scientists, and ethicists, is essential. By working together, these professionals can ensure the development of AI technologies that not only meet technological requirements but also align with the practical needs of clinicians and the ethical concerns of patients. Moreover, fostering partnerships between academia, industry, and healthcare institutions can drive forward research and development initiatives tailored to overcoming these technological challenges.

Continuous education and training are also crucial. Healthcare professionals must be equipped with the knowledge and skills to use AI technologies effectively in their practice. Regular training and upskilling can ensure that clinicians stay abreast of technological advancements, enhancing their ability to interact with AI-driven systems confidently and competently. Creating educational programs focused on AI's role in medicine that are accessible to both current practitioners and future generations can lay the groundwork for smoother technological integration.

Finally, there's the concern of costs associated with AI implementation. While AI promises long-term cost savings through increased efficiency and precision, the initial costs of infrastructure upgrades, training, and development can be a significant barrier, especially for resource-limited healthcare providers. Governments, policymakers, and organizations can play a role here by providing financial incentives and support for AI adoption in healthcare. This support can include funding for research, subsidies for infrastructure development, or tax incentives for institutions willing to adopt AI technologies.

Despite these challenges, the trajectory of AI in medicine is poised for growth. With targeted efforts to overcome technological barriers, the healthcare industry can not only harness the power of AI to improve patient outcomes, but it can also lead the way in creating a more sustainable, efficient, and effective system of care. The journey towards fully integrating AI in medicine is undoubtedly complex, yet with determination and collaboration, it is entirely achievable.

Navigating Regulatory Landscapes

The promise of artificial intelligence in medicine is vast, teeming with potential to revolutionize diagnostics, treatment, and patient care. However, even the most advanced technologies face a dynamic landscape of regulations that greatly influences their implementation. Navigating these regulatory terrains is a challenge unto itself, layered with complexities and inconsistencies across different regions.

Understanding these landscapes is crucial for innovators eager to integrate AI into the heart of healthcare.

Regulations are pivotal in ensuring the safety and efficacy of AI applications in healthcare. They create frameworks within which technologies can be safely deployed, protecting patients from potential harm. Yet, these same safeguards often raise barriers to innovation and slow the introduction of new AI tools. As such, developers and healthcare providers must balance the stringent requirements with innovative deployment strategies. This balance is not always easy to achieve, and it requires a careful orchestration of compliance and creativity.

The regulatory environment for AI in medicine is still evolving, playing catch-up with the rapid pace of technological advances. Unlike traditional medical devices, AI systems possess an inherent capacity for learning and evolving, challenging existing approval processes that focus primarily on static products. Current regulations may not fully account for AI's adaptive nature, prompting a shift towards new frameworks that can better accommodate continuous learning algorithms. This dynamic presents a unique challenge: how to regulate AI systems that change and improve over time?

One central consideration in the regulatory process is the classification of AI tools as medical devices. Whether an AI application falls under such a classification typically dictates the intensity of scrutiny and requirements for market entry. This classification is not always straightforward. For example, an AI-driven app that provides general health advice might not be scrutinized as strictly as an AI system intended to diagnose diseases. This ambiguity can sometimes create a gray area for developers trying to navigate regulatory channels. Clearer guidelines and classifications are needed to aid the development process and ensure that AI tools are appropriately vetted.

The role of data in AI systems cannot be overstated, and with it comes the challenge of data privacy and security. Regulations like the Health Insurance Portability and Accountability Act (HIPAA) in the United States and the General Data Protection Regulation (GDPR) in Europe set strict rules on how patient data can be used. These rules ensure that individual privacy is protected, but they also add complexity to the development and deployment of AI systems. Meeting these regulatory requirements requires a robust framework for data governance, which is essential for gaining trust from both regulators and the public.

International disparities in regulations create additional hurdles. AI solutions developed in one country often must undergo a separate series of approvals to be authorized elsewhere, leading to potential delays in availability and increased development costs. Countries are currently working to bridge these gaps through harmonization efforts, aiming to create more cohesive international standards. However, these efforts are still in their infancy, and achieving true regulatory congruence is a long-term endeavor.

Another area of significant regulatory importance is the transparency and explainability of AI algorithms. Patients and practitioners need to understand how AI systems reach their conclusions, especially when those conclusions impact critical medical decisions. Regulators emphasize the necessity of explainable AI, where the decision-making process should be interpretable to ensure accountability and enhance trust. Developing AI technologies with such transparency in mind is an ongoing challenge that requires addressing complex technical issues and reforming current practices.

In some cases, traditional regulatory frameworks may be ill-suited to the fast-paced nature of AI development. Regulators are beginning to consider more agile approaches, such as "sandbox" environments, where AI technologies can be tested safely in real-world settings without full regulatory approval. These environments allow regulators and developers to collaborate directly, fostering innovation while ensuring patient safety. Such initiatives point towards a more collaborative future where regulatory processes are as dynamic and adaptable as AI technologies themselves.

Engaging with policymakers early and often in the development process is crucial for navigating regulatory barriers. This engagement not only aids compliance but also helps shape policies that are more aligned with the realities of AI in healthcare. Active participation in policy development by AI innovators ensures that regulations evolve in a way that is conducive to technological advancement without compromising patient safety or ethical standards.

Looking ahead, the landscape is likely to become more navigable as regulators gain deeper insights and experience with AI technologies. Continued dialogue between technologists, healthcare providers, and regulatory bodies will be essential in crafting guidelines that protect the public while fostering innovation. As more AI applications prove their worth in healthcare settings, there will be increased momentum towards refining and streamlining regulatory processes.

Ultimately, navigating the regulatory landscape is not just a matter of overcoming obstacles; it's about ensuring that as AI transforms medicine, it does so in a manner that is safe, ethical, and beneficial for all. Embracing the challenge of regulation can lead to more robust and well-tested solutions, creating a healthcare environment where technology and regulation work hand in hand for the betterment of patient care.

Chapter 21:
The Future of AI in Precision Medicine

The future of AI in precision medicine stands on the cusp of transformative change, promising a new era in healthcare where treatment isn't just personalized but anticipates patients' needs with unprecedented accuracy. Imagine a world where AI not only suggests tailored therapies based on an individual's genetic makeup but predicts potential health risks with a level of precision that allows for preemptive intervention. This is becoming a reality as visionary projects push the boundaries of what's possible, integrating AI into everyday practice to deliver care that's not just reactive but proactive. The key lies in synthesizing vast datasets, from genomics to real-time health metrics, enabling clinicians to craft bespoke treatment plans that evolve with the patient. As AI continues to mature, its seamless incorporation into daily clinical workflows will redefine patient care, unlocking possibilities that are only beginning to unfold. Balancing innovation with ethical considerations will be crucial, as we aim to harness AI's potential for the ultimate goal: better health outcomes for all. Precision medicine, once an ambitious concept, is rapidly becoming a cornerstone of tomorrow's healthcare, driven by the relentless advancements in AI technology.

Visionary Projects and Expectations

The future of AI in precision medicine is not merely about what's on the horizon; it's about reimagining the very essence of healthcare. As we stand at the cusp of this new era, visionary projects are already set in motion, aiming to revolutionize patient care in innovative and profound ways. These projects don't just push the boundaries of what's possible—they redefine them, drawing from cutting-edge technologies and ground-breaking research.

In recent years, there have been remarkable strides in leveraging AI to create highly personalized treatment plans. Researchers and tech companies are focusing on building AI systems that can analyze extensive datasets, from genomic sequences to electronic health records, to predict an individual's response to certain treatments. The implications of such projects are profound. Imagine a world where AI could provide a personalized health roadmap for each person, optimizing therapeutic strategies, minimizing adverse effects, and significantly enhancing treatment outcomes. This is not science fiction; it is becoming an emerging reality.

Among these visionary projects is the ongoing development of AI algorithms capable of simulating clinical trials. Instead of traditional methods, which are time-consuming and costly, these AI-driven virtual trials can model biological interactions and predict the efficacy of drugs quickly and with much less resource allocation. This approach not only accelerates the drug discovery process but also democratizes access to trial results, offering insights into the feasibility of personalizing drug combinations based on genetic markers and environmental factors.

Predictive analytics using AI in detecting potential outbreaks and drug shortages is yet another exciting development. These systems are designed to study patterns in health data, providing early warnings that can save lives and resources. An AI system that predicts a potential influenza outbreak based on real-time data from wearable technologies could revolutionize public health responses. It's about transitioning from reactive to proactive healthcare, offering a foresight-driven approach that protects populations from emerging health threats.

Additionally, AI-powered platforms are being developed to facilitate seamless data exchange among patients, healthcare providers, and researchers across the globe. Interoperability remains a significant challenge in the current healthcare framework, but with AI, there is potential for creating a more integrated system. These platforms could lead to global health solutions that understand the subtle nuances of disease and health determinants across demographics, paving the way for universal standards in personalized care.

Consider, for instance, the vision of AI mentors in medical education, designed to closely mimic human insight and guidance. These advanced AI tools can provide personalized tutoring to medical students, validating their clinical reasoning with real-time feedback based on a vast repository of medical knowledge and case studies. Such technologies have the potential to cultivate a generation of healthcare professionals who are more prepared, more informed, and more compassionate in their practice.

In clinics and hospitals, AI is anticipated to take on a more prominent role, complementing healthcare teams and augmenting diagnostic processes. AI systems could provide second opinions on complex cases, assist with surgical procedures by precisely mapping out surgical plans, and even help manage hospital logistics to enhance patient throughput. This integration aims not just at efficiency but at creating an environment where healthcare providers can focus more on patient-centered care.

Equally inspiring are collaborations between tech giants and healthcare pioneers, working towards AI-driven public health initiatives in underserved regions. AI has the unique capability of scaling solutions and bridging gaps in healthcare access. Projects aimed at developing low-cost diagnosis tools powered by AI can bring medical insight to the remotest corners of the world, empowering communities with solutions that were once limited to well-equipped urban centers.

To truly harness the full potential of AI in precision medicine, we must also consider the ethical dimensions. Ensuring that these transformative tools are developed responsibly requires addressing biases in AI algorithms and upholding stringent data privacy measures. This is a critical focus area for forward-thinking projects designing AI systems that are not just technologically advanced but also ethically sound and universally fair.

The expectations surrounding AI in precision medicine are undeniably high and, while challenges lie ahead, the prospects of integrating AI into routine healthcare practice are boundless. Visionaries in the field urge a rethinking of regulatory frameworks to support rapid advancements while ensuring patient safety. Institutions are crafting guidelines to strike a balance between innovation and oversight, encouraging responsible yet breakthrough-driven progress.

Ultimately, the future of AI in precision medicine is about realizing a vision where healthcare is not only advanced but also personalized, accessible, and sustainable. These visionary projects pave the way for a transformative impact, promising a future where AI becomes an indispensable ally in our quest for health and longevity. As we step forward, we carry the hope that these technological wonders will usher us into an era of enhanced human health and well-being, making science fiction an everyday reality.

Integrating AI into Everyday Practice

Integrating artificial intelligence into the everyday practice of precision medicine stands as one of the most profound transformations in contemporary healthcare. As AI technologies evolve, they aren't just tools—they're becoming partners in patient care. This reshaping of medical practice doesn't happen in a vacuum; it requires a seamless blending of advanced algorithms with the human touch that characterizes effective healthcare. The path to this integration is paved with both challenges and opportunities, yet the potential benefits make the journey not only worthwhile but necessary.

One of the essential components of integrating AI into routine practice is the development of intuitive interfaces for healthcare professionals. These interfaces need to be user-friendly to enable practitioners to focus on patient care rather than wrestling with complex algorithms. Here, the design of AI systems becomes crucial— systems should complement rather than complicate the physician's workflow. Imagine a scenario where a doctor can assess a patient's genetic data and lifestyle information within minutes, allowing for a tailored treatment plan that is both quick and highly personalized. This is no longer a distant vision, but a burgeoning reality.

The introduction of AI into everyday clinical decisions creates opportunities for improving accuracy and efficiency. AI can evaluate vast amounts of data at speeds inconceivable to the human mind, identifying patterns and anomalies that might elude even the most experienced clinicians. For instance, AI can rapidly process medical images, offering second opinions almost instantaneously and with great precision. This kind of assistance can be particularly valuable in areas where diagnostic errors might lead to significant consequences.

Moreover, AI's role in predictive analytics is a leap towards proactive rather than reactive healthcare. By analyzing historical data alongside real-time inputs, AI can identify potential health crises before they manifest, allowing for early intervention. For example, predicting a patient's likelihood of developing a chronic disease based on lifestyle habits, genetics, and environmental factors is increasingly feasible. Early warnings can lead to lifestyle adjustments that might prevent the disease altogether, significantly enhancing quality of life and reducing healthcare costs.

This seamless integration does not stop at diagnostics and predictions—it extends to enabling personalized communication between healthcare providers and patients. AI-powered platforms can distill complex medical information into patient-friendly insights, promoting better understanding and adherence to prescribed treatments. With AI, the delivery of healthcare information becomes a two-way street, empowering patients by keeping them informed and engaged in their health journey.

A crucial aspect of embedding AI into everyday practice is continuous learning and adaptability. AI systems aren't static; they're designed to learn from each interaction, becoming increasingly refined over time. This potential for growth suggests a future where AI systems provide not only medical insights but also personalized recommendations tailored to individual preferences and needs. These capabilities could transform patient management, encouraging a much-needed shift towards personalized medicine.

The integration of AI also offers remarkable benefits in the realm of telemedicine, fueling a transformation already underway. AI technologies can assist in conducting remote examinations, improving accessibility to specialized care regardless of geographical barriers. In rural or underserved areas, AI-driven virtual consultations could ensure that patients receive timely and accurate medical advice, significantly expanding the reach of healthcare services.

Yet, alongside these advancements, there's a need for careful consideration of ethical and regulatory frameworks. As AI becomes ever more present in healthcare ecosystems, privacy and security issues come to the forefront. Protecting patient data from breaches while allowing for the immense analytical power of AI requires robust security measures and clear regulatory guidelines. Creating a balance between technological advancements and ethical considerations is paramount to maintaining public trust.

Successful integration also hinges on continuous education and collaboration. It requires that healthcare providers remain informed about AI capabilities, limitations, and updates. Multidisciplinary collaboration among technologists, ethicists, clinicians, and policymakers is essential in navigating the complexities AI introduces. By cultivating a culture of collaboration and learning, the medical community can harness the full potential of AI while minimizing its drawbacks.

As AI becomes more entrenched in medical practice, it also amplifies the need for empathy in healthcare. While AI can analyze data and provide insights, it doesn't replace the essential human elements of medicine—compassion, empathy, and understanding. Physicians using AI must remember their critical role in interpreting and communicating this intelligence. Empathy should remain central in all patient interactions, ensuring that technology serves as an aid, not a replacement, in nurturing patient trust and comfort.

Looking towards the future, integrating AI into everyday practice will undoubtedly redefine the physician's role. Conceivably, doctors will transition from data analysts to health strategists, focusing more on patient interaction and less on the minutiae of data interpretation. As AI takes on more background analytical tasks, physicians will have the opportunity to spend more meaningful time with their patients, fostering deeper relationships and more tailored healthcare strategies.

In conclusion, the integration of AI into everyday practice in precision medicine does not simply alter the logistics of healthcare—it reimagines its very fabric. This integration signals a future where AI and healthcare professionals coalesce seamlessly, each amplifying the other's strengths. By leveraging these technologies judiciously, the medical community has the potential to enhance patient care in ways previously thought impossible. The journey may be challenging, requiring careful navigation of technological, ethical, and human factors, but the destination—a more connected, efficient, and personalized healthcare experience—is well worth the effort.

Chapter 22:
AI's Role in Elderly Care

As the global population ages, there's an increasing need for innovative solutions to cater to the unique healthcare requirements of older adults, and artificial intelligence is stepping up to meet this challenge. AI technologies are being designed to not only monitor health conditions but also predict potential medical issues before they manifest, offering a level of proactive care that was previously unimaginable. Consider AI-powered home assistants that remind the elderly to take their medications, or smart wearable devices that track vital signs around the clock, alerting caregivers if something seems amiss. These tools aim to increase autonomy for seniors, allowing them to age gracefully in their own homes while providing peace of mind to their families. Furthermore, AI is helping in personalizing care plans to suit individual needs, ensuring that every aspect of a senior's health, from nutrition to mental well-being, is attentively managed. By integrating AI into elderly care, we're fostering an environment where aging is not just about managing decline, but enriching the later stages of life with dignity and safety.

Innovations for Aging Populations

As the global population ages, the need for innovative solutions in elderly care becomes more pressing. AI has emerged as a potent tool, transforming how we address the needs of aging individuals. It isn't just about living longer; it's about improving the quality of those additional years. With AI, we can implement more tailored, efficient, and compassionate care for the elderly.

One of the most significant contributions of AI in this field is the development of smart home technologies. These aren't just fancy gadgets; they're vital tools that help seniors maintain independence. AI-driven systems can monitor daily activities, notice deviations from routine that might indicate health issues, and even learn to predict potential problems before they occur. For example, AI can monitor a senior's gait and identify changes that could signal an increased risk of falls. Through this kind of subtle surveillance, families and caregivers gain peace of mind, knowing that they will be alerted to any troubling changes in behavior.

AI-powered personal assistants are another boon for older adults. These devices, equipped with natural language processing, can engage in conversations, set reminders for medication, and even summon help in emergencies. Unlike traditional alert systems that require manual activation, AI assistants can be trained to recognize distress or incoherent speech patterns, triggering a call for help automatically. Beyond providing immediate assistance, these systems can also alleviate feelings of isolation by maintaining a form of social interaction.

Telemedicine, augmented by AI, has already proven invaluable in reaching older adults, especially those with limited mobility. AI-enhanced diagnostics and consultations offer quick and precise assessments. Seniors can engage in comprehensive healthcare assessments without leaving their homes, which is particularly beneficial during inclement weather or when traveling is difficult. Moreover, AI can continuously analyze patient data over time, providing healthcare providers with a more comprehensive picture of a patient's health, facilitating early intervention.

Wearable technology, embedded with AI, is also taking the lead. Devices like smartwatches that track heart rate, sleep patterns, and physical activity can now offer insights far beyond data collection. AI algorithms interpret this data to alert both seniors and caregivers about unusual trends or activities. For instance, a sudden drop in physical activity might indicate health issues that require attention, allowing preemptive measures rather than reactive treatments.

Moreover, AI provides breakthroughs in personalized nutrition and exercise regimens for the elderly. Customization is crucial because nutritional needs change with age, as do responses to physical activity. AI systems can recommend dietary adjustments and exercise routines tailored to an individual's health history and current condition. This personalization helps enhance the overall well-being of seniors, addressing specific metabolic changes, medication interactions, and other age-related factors.

From a different perspective, AI supports caregivers too. It reduces the burden by taking over repetitive monitoring tasks, thus allowing human caregivers to focus on relationship-based care. Emotional and psychological support for caregivers, often overlooked, is more feasible when AI shoulders some of the load. Tools that analyze caregiver stress levels and workload can suggest interventions to prevent burnout, ensuring the longevity and quality of care provided to seniors.

One of the more innovative uses of AI in elderly care is through virtual reality (VR) and augmented reality (AR). These technologies, powered by AI, open new avenues for cognitive training and social engagement. For seniors dealing with dementia or cognitive decline, VR experiences can help stimulate memory and cognitive function. For others, virtual travel or social activities foster a sense of engagement and community, which is vital in reducing the loneliness epidemic among the elderly.

AI-piloted robots are finding roles in elderly care as well. More than just futuristic toys, these robots can assist with daily tasks like meal preparation, cleaning, and even medical administration. They can also facilitate communication with far-away family members through video calls, making frequent check-ins possible without the need for someone to be physically present. These robots are designed to be user-friendly, requiring minimal learning time for the elderly, and making them accessible aids rather than technological barriers.

Furthermore, AI is pioneering early disease detection in the aging population. Predictive analytics tools process vast datasets to identify patterns indicative of conditions such as Alzheimer's or Parkinson's long before symptoms are evident. This early detection is crucial because it allows for interventions that can significantly alter the disease's course, enhancing quality of life and potentially prolonging it.

The integration of AI in medication management is another critical advancement. With automated systems tracking prescriptions, reminding users when to take their medication, and even dispensing the correct dosages, the challenge of adherence is markedly reduced. These systems can adapt to changes in a medical regimen swiftly, ensuring accuracy and safety for patients with complex medication schedules.

In the broader healthcare ecosystem, AI helps streamline the transition from hospital to home care, coordinating with various health professionals to ensure continuity of care. For older adults, this can mean a seamless transition, fewer readmissions, and effective long-term health management, which is key to aging gracefully at home.

Adapting AI innovations for the aging population offers incredible promise. As technology continues to evolve, we can expect AI to further revolutionize elderly care, ensuring not just longer lives, but more fulfilling ones. While challenges remain, particularly in ensuring accessibility and managing ethical concerns, the potential benefits AI brings in enhancing the lives of the elderly are immense and inspiring. The ultimate goal is a world where aging is met with dignity, understanding, and support, facilitated significantly by the intelligent use of AI.

AI Tools for Enhanced Elder Care

The integration of AI in elder care represents not just a leap in technological advancement, but a compassionate step forward in enhancing the quality of life for aging populations. At the heart of this transformation are AI tools designed to meet the unique challenges that come with aging. As people live longer, the demand for effective, efficient, and empathetic elder care solutions is more pressing than ever. AI is stepping up, offering tools that can assist in everything from daily living to advanced medical care, ensuring that the elderly can lead dignified and fulfilling lives.

One of the most significant areas where AI is making a difference is through the use of smart assistants and home automation systems. These systems, often integrated with AI-powered voice recognition and learning capabilities, can help seniors manage daily tasks. Whether it's reminding them to take medications, assisting with grocery orders, or even providing companionship through conversation, these AI companions lend a supportive hand. Through natural language processing, these tools evolve, learning preferences and patterns to provide personalized experiences and comfort.

AI tools are also revolutionizing personal safety for seniors living at home. Wearable devices and sensors equipped with AI capabilities can monitor movement and vital signs, detecting falls or other medical emergencies. These systems can alert emergency services or designated caregivers, allowing for swift intervention. The peace of mind provided to both seniors and their families cannot be overstated. With real-time monitoring and predictive analytics, potential health issues can be flagged before they escalate, enabling preventive measures that enhance both safety and longevity.

In the realm of healthcare management, AI plays a crucial role in coordinating complex care needs. Elderly patients often juggle multiple healthcare providers, medications, and treatment plans. AI systems can synthesize data from various sources to create comprehensive care logs, offering insights that help healthcare professionals make informed decisions. This level of integration ensures consistent and coherent care, minimizing the risk of adverse drug interactions and improving health outcomes.

Furthermore, AI is proving invaluable in cognitive health management. With its capacity to analyze large datasets, AI can assist in early detection and intervention strategies for cognitive decline. By evaluating speech patterns, facial expressions, and other subtle behavioral cues, AI can offer insights into the progression of dementia-related conditions. Early diagnosis alerts families and health professionals to intervene sooner, possibly slowing disease progression with appropriate therapies and lifestyle adjustments.

In addition, the convenience of AI-driven telehealth services cannot be overlooked. For those with mobility issues or those living in remote areas, virtual consultations conducted through AI-enhanced platforms provide critical access to medical expertise without the need for travel. These platforms can perform preliminary assessments, organize patient data for specialists, and even facilitate routine check-ins—making healthcare more accessible and comprehensive for elders.

AI-driven innovations are also revolutionizing physical rehabilitation. Intelligent robots and AI systems assist in guided exercises tailored to individual abilities. By analyzing real-time data, these tools provide adaptive feedback, helping elders regain physical strength and mobility. This approach not only enhances recovery times but also fosters a sense of independence and motivation among elderly users.

AI's role in elder care extends to mental health. Social isolation is a prevalent issue among older adults, leading to depression and anxiety. AI-based applications that use virtual reality or interactive storytelling can significantly combat these feelings by providing immersive experiences that stimulate mental engagement and social interaction. Such tools help maintain mental acuity while fostering a sense of connection to the broader world.

Moreover, AI tools are invaluable in resource management within senior living environments. They can manage and optimize logistics, from scheduling staff shifts to inventorying supplies, ensuring that resources are used efficiently. This optimization allows caregivers to focus more on personal interactions and less on administrative burdens, directly enhancing the quality of care received by residents.

In conclusion, AI tools for elder care not only meet the practical needs of an aging population but also address their emotional and psychological well-being. By fostering environments where seniors feel supported, empowered, and secure, AI is helping redefine aging. As technology advances, it's crucial to maintain an ethical focus, ensuring that AI remains a force for good—one that respects the dignity and individuality of every elderly person. Embracing these innovations offers a promising path forward, transforming elder care into an arena where compassion and technology harmoniously coexist.

Chapter 23:
AI in Pediatrics

As we transition into exploring AI's transformative role in pediatrics, we see a landscape ripe with potential for improving child health management and specialized care. With AI, pediatricians now have robust tools to delve deeper into developmental health, often with a precision previously unattainable. Innovative applications in predictive analytics help foresee potential health issues in children, enabling preemptive action and individualized treatment plans. AI aids in deciphering complex pediatric conditions like congenital heart defects and rare genetic disorders where early diagnosis and intervention are crucial. The technology complements traditional care, not replacing the irreplaceable human touch but rather enhancing it, ensuring every child's unique needs are met with a blend of compassion and cutting-edge technology. While challenges remain, such as ensuring algorithm fairness and safeguarding sensitive data, the horizon is bright. This evolving synergy between AI and pediatrics promises a new era where young lives can thrive, nurtured by insights and care backed by advanced science.

Advancements in Child Health Management

The transformative power of artificial intelligence (AI) is palpable across the medical spectrum, but nowhere is its impact more promising than in the realm of child health management. Children, with their unique physiological and developmental needs, pose a distinct challenge in healthcare. AI is stepping in to meet this challenge by providing innovative solutions that offer hope for healthier generations.

One of the critical areas AI is making strides in is early diagnosis and intervention. Children's health issues, if caught early, can often be managed or even reversed, leading to vastly improved life outcomes. With predictive analytics, AI can sift through vast amounts of data, including genetics, family history, and environmental factors, to identify children at risk of developing certain conditions. For instance, algorithms have been developed to predict the likelihood of developing autism spectrum disorders by analyzing subtle patterns in behavior and communication. This early detection allows healthcare providers to intervene promptly, deploying therapies and support systems that have the biggest impact when started early.

Moreover, AI is transforming the management of chronic conditions in children. Asthma, diabetes, and epilepsy are just a few examples of chronic conditions that affect children's lives profoundly. AI-powered monitoring devices and applications provide continuous real-time data, enabling personalized care and timely interventions. These systems can alert caregivers of a child's deteriorating condition before it becomes critical, thus averting hospitalizations and enhancing the child's quality of life. Similarly, AI models can analyze various data points from a child's interactions with healthcare devices to adjust treatment regimens dynamically, ensuring that each child receives the most effective care tailored to their ongoing needs.

In pediatric care, communication with young patients and their families is crucial for effective treatment. AI's role as a communication facilitator can't be underestimated. Through natural language processing and conversational interfaces, AI-powered platforms can enhance patient-doctor communication, breaking down complex medical language into information that's accessible and understandable for both children and their parents. This empowers families to take a more informed and active role in managing their child's health.

AI is also making waves in the field of personalized medicine for children. By integrating data from various sources like electronic health records and genomic data, AI systems can develop highly personalized treatment plans that account for a child's unique biological makeup. This capability is particularly beneficial in pediatrics, where traditional "one-size-fits-all" treatments are often less effective. For example, in pediatric oncology, AI has been used to tailor chemotherapies that optimize efficacy while minimizing side effects, providing a critical advantage in treating young patients whose bodies are still developing.

The role of AI extends beyond treatment to the realm of preventive healthcare and wellness management. AI systems can model the potential impact of lifestyle changes on a child's current and future health, providing actionable insights for caregivers. This proactivity in health management encourages good health practices from a young age, setting the foundation for healthier adulthood.

Furthermore, AI is redefining how pediatric research is conducted. Traditionally, insights are derived from studying aggregated data from adults and then adapting those findings to treat children. However, AI enables the use of machine learning algorithms to rapidly analyze data specifically from pediatric populations, leading to discoveries that are not biased by adult-centric models. This child-specific research is already paving the way for new treatments that are bespoke to the delicacies of juvenile physiology.

Ethical considerations remain at the forefront as AI continues to permeate pediatric healthcare. Ensuring data privacy and consenting practices suitable for younger patients are crucial ethical challenges that accompany technological advancements. By establishing robust ethical frameworks and engaging parents, caregivers, and children themselves where appropriate, these concerns can be addressed effectively, fostering trust in AI systems.

Finally, it's essential not to overlook the role of AI in supporting caregivers and healthcare professionals. The administrative load that comes with pediatric care can be taxing; AI aids in streamlining these tasks. From automating routine paperwork to optimizing appointment scheduling, AI frees up medical professionals to concentrate more on patient care, thereby enhancing overall healthcare delivery.

The journey of integrating AI into pediatric health management is just beginning, yet its potential to revolutionize this field is undeniable. As AI technology continues to evolve, it promises not only to change how we treat and manage children's health issues today but also to reshape the very landscape of pediatric healthcare for future generations. By harnessing AI responsibly and creatively, we can look forward to a future where our youngest members of society receive care that's not only smarter and more efficient but also profoundly compassionate and intuitively responsive to their unique needs.

AI Applications for Pediatric Specialties

The field of pediatrics is uniquely challenging, owing to the dynamic physiological, psychological, and developmental stages children go through. AI applications are emerging as transformative tools within this specialty, offering new avenues for enhancing diagnosis, treatment, and monitoring child health conditions. As we pivot towards the integration of AI in pediatric specialties, it becomes evident that the technology's potential hinges on its ability to adapt to the nuanced needs of this demographic. From neonatal care to adolescent medicine, AI is proving itself an invaluable ally in pediatric healthcare.

One of the standout applications of AI in pediatrics lies in the area of neonatal care. Newborns, especially those in neonatal intensive care units (NICUs), require constant monitoring due to their vulnerability to a plethora of health issues. AI-driven devices can continuously analyze data from a newborn's vital signs, including heart rate, oxygen levels, and respiration. This real-time monitoring allows for the early detection of potential health issues such as respiratory distress or sepsis. By promptly alerting healthcare providers to subtle changes in a baby's condition, AI systems facilitate timely interventions, which can be critical in preventing complications or improving outcomes.

Moreover, AI is revolutionizing pediatric cardiology by offering precise diagnostic support for congenital heart defects (CHDs), which are among the most common types of birth defects. Traditional diagnostic methods like echocardiograms, while effective, can be time-consuming and dependent on the expertise of the clinician. AI algorithms, trained on vast datasets, can assist in interpreting echocardiograms with a remarkable degree of accuracy. These systems can help identify CHDs more efficiently and at an earlier stage, leading to more proactive and targeted treatment strategies.

Pediatric oncology is another specialty witnessing a significant impact from AI advancements. By analyzing complex data from genomic sequencing and clinical trials, AI tools can predict cancer progression and response to treatment options in young patients. This predictive capability supports the personalization of cancer therapies, ensuring that treatments are not only more effective but also minimize potential side effects commonly experienced by children. The ability to tailor cancer therapies based on a child's unique genetic makeup represents a monumental step toward more compassionate and responsive pediatric care.

In pediatric neurology, AI applications are being explored to enhance the diagnosis and management of neurological disorders such as epilepsy and autism spectrum disorders (ASDs). For instance, machine learning models can analyze electroencephalography (EEG) data to help predict seizures in epileptic children, giving caregivers and medical professionals a critical heads-up before an event occurs. Similarly, AI can aid in the early detection of ASDs by processing vast amounts of behavioral data, which can be instrumental in initiating early intervention strategies crucial to long-term outcomes.

AI's role in pediatric endocrinology is particularly noteworthy in the management of type 1 diabetes. With AI-powered continuous glucose monitoring systems and insulin pumps, young patients and their families can manage blood sugar levels more effectively. These devices use machine learning to predict glucose trends, adjust insulin delivery, and provide real-time recommendations, thus empowering children to lead more normal and active lives. Such innovations reduce the burden on caregivers and significantly enhance the quality of life for diabetic children.

In the context of pediatric pulmonology, AI applications are enhancing the management of respiratory conditions like asthma. AI algorithms can analyze environmental data, patient history, and symptom patterns to predict asthma attacks or exacerbations. By alerting both patients and healthcare providers to potential risks, these applications enable more proactive management of the condition, potentially reducing hospital visits and improving overall patient outcomes.

AI's impact on pediatric specialties extends to improving surgical outcomes. Pediatric surgeries often involve distinct challenges given the smaller anatomical structures and variable physiological responses of children. Robotics and AI-assisted technologies offer unprecedented precision and control in surgical procedures. They can also simulate and plan complex surgeries, leading to reduced surgical times and faster recoveries. Furthermore, AI-driven platforms provide surgical training and decision support, which are vital in developing pediatric surgeons' expertise.

The educational aspect of pediatric healthcare and how AI can support young patients' understanding of their conditions shouldn't be overlooked. Interactive AI tools are being developed to educate children about their diagnoses, treatment plans, and health management in an engaging and accessible manner. By utilizing gamification and augmented reality, these tools aim to demystify medical processes and empower children to become active participants in their own healthcare journeys.

While AI in pediatric specialties offers numerous benefits, it also raises important ethical and practical considerations. The sensitivity of children's health data demands rigorous privacy and security measures. Ensuring AI systems are free from bias and are designed with inclusivity in mind is crucial to avoid disparities in care. Additionally, fostering trust among parents and pediatricians in AI tools is essential for their widespread adoption and optimal implementation.

In conclusion, AI is rapidly becoming an indispensable tool in pediatric specialties, enhancing the precision and efficacy of healthcare delivery for children. As AI technology continues to evolve, its applications within pediatrics will likely expand, offering innovative solutions to longstanding challenges. The promise of AI in this field lies in its ability to not only improve clinical outcomes but also promote a more personalized, compassionate, and informed healthcare experience for our youngest patients.

Chapter 24:
Public Perception of AI in Healthcare

As artificial intelligence steadily permeates the healthcare landscape, public perception plays a pivotal role in shaping its trajectory. While AI holds incredible promise—ranging from enhancing diagnostic accuracy to crafting personalized treatment plans—it's met with a mix of anticipation and skepticism. Trust in AI's capabilities depends on transparency and the communication of its benefits and limitations to the broader public. Fostering understanding through education and dialogue can bridge the gap between innovation and apprehension, promoting trust and acceptance. As patients and medical professionals gain more firsthand experience with AI, misconceptions often give way to recognition of its potential to transform care. The journey toward widespread endorsement of AI in healthcare isn't without challenges, but through collaborative effort and continued advancement, the public's embrace seems a hopeful inevitability.

Understanding Societal Views

As artificial intelligence increasingly finds its footing in healthcare, understanding how society perceives this transformation is crucial. People's views on AI in healthcare form a complex tapestry woven from optimism, skepticism, fear, and curiosity. This section delves into these varied perceptions, exploring the factors that shape them and the consequences they may have on AI adoption and healthcare outcomes.

At the heart of societal views on AI in healthcare is the promise of enhanced efficiency and effectiveness. Many see AI as a tool that could revolutionize diagnostics and treatment delivery, providing unprecedented accuracy and speed. For healthcare professionals facing increasing workloads, AI offers a potential remedy by shouldering some of the burdens associated with patient care. This promise of relief drives enthusiasm among medical communities eager to embrace cutting-edge solutions.

However, this optimism is not universally shared. Some members of the public harbor concerns about AI's role in healthcare, mainly revolving around its ethical and practical implications. High-profile cases of AI failures or biases in other sectors prompt questions about trustworthiness and reliability. People often worry about how machines might make life-altering decisions, prompting discussions about the potential risks versus the benefits AI presents in medical settings.

Cultural influences also play a pivotal role in shaping societal views on AI in healthcare. In many eastern countries, where technological integration is generally embraced, AI is perceived as an inevitable and positive step forward. In contrast, western societies sometimes exhibit more caution, influenced by broader debates on data privacy, autonomy, and control in technology use. This cultural dichotomy can affect how AI solutions are developed and implemented across different regions.

Trust in AI in healthcare is closely tied to transparency and understanding. People want to know how AI systems make decisions, particularly those affecting their personal health. Yet, the underlying algorithms and data processes often remain a "black box," making it difficult for non-specialists to grasp. Increasing efforts to demystify AI through public engagements and educational campaigns can help bridge this gap, fostering greater acceptance and understanding.

Media portrayal of AI in healthcare also significantly impacts public perceptions. News stories highlighting successful AI-assisted surgeries or groundbreaking diagnostic tools contribute positively. Still, sensationalized reports focusing on errors or ethical dilemmas can sow fear and doubt. Balanced and informative media coverage is essential to paint an accurate picture of AI's capabilities and limitations in healthcare settings.

Engagement with AI technologies in personal life further shades societal views. Those acquainted with AI through consumer technology like smartphones or smart home devices may have an easier time accepting its application in healthcare, seeing AI as an extension of its already beneficial utility. Conversely, individuals with limited digital exposure might approach AI in healthcare with more reserve, unfamiliar with the scope and potential of these advanced systems.

Interestingly, public discourse around AI in healthcare often intersects with discussions on broader healthcare system reforms. People wonder how AI might address systemic issues such as equitable access to services or healthcare affordability. While AI holds potential solutions, there's awareness that it could also exacerbate disparities if not carefully managed. This duality sometimes fuels both hope and concern regarding AI's role in future healthcare landscapes.

Societal views also encompass concerns about the human touch in healthcare. Patients value empathy, understanding, and personal interaction, attributes that machines struggle to replicate. There is apprehension that AI-driven automation might erode these critical aspects of care. Balancing AI capabilities with human elements remains a critical consideration for healthcare providers and technology developers alike.

Demographics, including age and education level, can influence how people perceive AI in healthcare. Younger generations, steeped in technology from an early age, are generally more receptive to AI innovations. Meanwhile, older individuals might show hesitancy due to unfamiliarity or skepticism about its impact on traditional methods of care. Educational initiatives aimed at demystifying AI across diverse age groups are essential for widespread acceptance.

The role of social media in shaping societal views shouldn't be underestimated. Platforms like Twitter, Facebook, and Instagram facilitate rapid information exchange, allowing viewpoints on AI in healthcare to proliferate quickly. While this can aid in spreading awareness, it also means misinformation can spread equally fast, requiring vigilance from both the public and healthcare communicators to ensure accuracy in shared content.

Ultimately, understanding societal views on AI in healthcare is about recognizing this intricate weave of hopes, fears, opportunities, and challenges. As AI continues to evolve, societal attitudes and perceptions will undoubtedly play a significant role in dictating its trajectory and impact in the healthcare domain. Engaging with these diverse views through open dialogue and education is key to fostering a landscape where AI can complement human expertise, driving healthcare innovation forward responsibly and inclusively.

Promoting Trust and Acceptance

As artificial intelligence carves its path into the intricate fabric of healthcare, nurturing public trust and fostering acceptance is paramount. Trust is the cornerstone of any transformative technology, particularly in an arena as sensitive and personal as healthcare. People entrust their well-being to medical professionals, and introducing AI into this relationship requires both cautious optimism and comprehensive education.

One facet of building trust is transparency. When healthcare providers utilize AI technologies, it's vital for them to be open about how these tools work, the outcomes they produce, and the data they use. Patients need to understand that AI can enhance diagnostic accuracy, identify potential treatment options, and offer personalized healthcare plans based on vast datasets that a human alone could not process. This transparency cultivates a sense of partnership, as individuals feel informed and involved in their healthcare journey.

Moreover, the perceived infallibility of machines can both create confidence and sow distrust. Acknowledging that AI systems, much like humans, can sometimes err helps maintain realistic expectations. These systems are designed to assist, not replace, human judgment. By clearly defining the role AI plays in diagnostics, treatment, and patient monitoring, patients and healthcare professionals can work together to strike a balance where AI complements human expertise, strengthening the overall healthcare experience.

Communication also plays a critical role in promoting acceptance. Healthcare providers must possess the skills to explain complex AI operations in layman's terms, ensuring patients aren't feeling overwhelmed or intimidated by tech jargon. Providing relatable analogies and addressing potential fears or misconceptions can help demystify AI, making it more approachable and less foreign. This open discourse can alleviate anxiety and build confidence in AI-enhanced care.

The ethical application of AI in healthcare must be at the forefront of trust-building efforts. Patients and the general public need assurances that AI technologies adhere to strict ethical guidelines, particularly regarding privacy and consent. With sensitive health data at stake, ensuring robust data protection measures are in place is critical. Institutions must communicate their commitment to safeguarding personal information, reinforcing that patient confidentiality remains a top priority despite technological advances.

Educational initiatives can bridge the gap between innovation and apprehension. Incorporating AI education into medical curriculums addresses concerns from the ground up, equipping future healthcare providers with the knowledge and skills to leverage AI confidently and ethically. For the general public, supported learning opportunities, such as workshops, webinars, and informational campaigns, can illuminate AI's role in shaping modern medicine. These educational endeavors both inform and inspire, fostering a culture that embraces AI's potential within healthcare.

Incorporating patient feedback into the development and deployment of AI technologies further enhances trust. By listening to patient experiences and concerns, AI developers and healthcare providers can refine their systems to better meet the needs and expectations of those who rely on them. This feedback loop not only improves AI applications but also empowers patients, offering them a voice in the evolution of their healthcare landscape.

Collaborative efforts between technologists, healthcare professionals, and policymakers are essential in establishing a unified approach to introducing AI in healthcare. These partnerships can facilitate the creation of standards and regulations that guide AI use, ensuring that all stakeholders are aligned in their objectives and methodologies. Such collaborations can lead to a cohesive strategy for maximizing AI's benefits while minimizing risks, thereby nurturing public trust and acceptance more effectively.

Another crucial element is showcasing success stories that highlight AI's positive impact on patient care. Real-life examples of AI improving diagnostic accuracy, enabling timely treatment interventions, and personalizing care plans can mute skepticism and inspire confidence. These stories humanize technology, transforming abstract concepts into tangible improvements in health outcomes that resonate with the public.

Ultimately, promoting trust and acceptance of AI in healthcare hinges on a multifaceted approach that combines transparency, education, ethical practices, and patient engagement. As AI continues to revolutionize the medical field, its integration into healthcare ecosystems must be handled with care and consideration, ensuring that innovation is harmonized with empathy and patient-centered care. Through these efforts, AI can become not only a symbol of technological progress but also a trusted ally in enhancing human health and well-being.

Chapter 25:
AI Innovations Beyond the Hospital

As we venture beyond the hospital walls, artificial intelligence opens a frontier where community health flourishes through collaboration and innovation. In this new landscape, AI technologies are redefining preventive care, providing remote monitoring tools that empower individuals to take charge of their health with unprecedented precision. Imagine AI-driven systems in communities, designed to detect early signs of health issues, offering guidance and intervention long before traditional models would allow. These advancements aren't just futuristic dreams—they're becoming vital in public health initiatives, where predictive analytics provide invaluable insights to health organizations, enabling them to allocate resources efficiently and address imminent health threats before they take root. As AI continues to seep into the everyday fabric of community wellness, it's reshaping the societal approach to health from reactive to proactive, enhancing the overall quality of life and democratizing access to healthcare resources. By fostering a connection between advanced technology and community well-being, AI is not just changing healthcare—it's changing lives, one community at a time.

Community Health Opportunities

The transformative power of artificial intelligence (AI) extends far beyond the walls of hospitals and clinics, permeating into communities to redefine how we approach public health. This shift is not merely

172

about redefining healthcare access; it's about harnessing AI to build healthier communities from the ground up. By analyzing vast amounts of data and spotting trends in real time, AI holds the promise to predict health outbreaks, personalize community health initiatives, and optimize resource distribution.

One of the most promising aspects of AI in community health is its ability to predict and prevent disease outbreaks. AI algorithms can sift through diverse datasets, including weather patterns, social media feeds, and population movement statistics, to detect potential health crises before they emerge. Imagine a system that alerts communities about a rising flu trend or predicts the next hotspot for a virus outbreak. These predictive capabilities enable public health officials to initiate early interventions, organize vaccine drives, and educate populations on preventive measures, thereby potentially saving countless lives.

But AI's role doesn't stop at prediction. Personalized health interventions at the community level are becoming a reality, thanks to AI's data-processing power. Tailoring health campaigns to the specific needs and behaviors of a community can drastically improve their effectiveness. AI can analyze the demographic distributions, prevalent health issues, and even cultural preferences of a community to design custom health initiatives. For example, an AI-driven platform could assess a neighborhood's dietary habits and suggest targeted nutrition workshops or healthy food access programs that resonate with residents.

Moreover, AI-powered tools are revolutionizing how we track and manage chronic diseases in communities. Wearable devices and mobile apps equipped with AI can monitor individual health metrics—such as blood sugar levels or heart rate—providing continuous and personalized feedback. These tools not only empower individuals to manage their health proactively but also enable healthcare providers to access aggregated data that highlights broader community health trends. This real-time data collection helps in the formulation of local policies and interventions better aligned with the actual needs of the population.

Resource allocation, a perennial challenge in public health, is also benefiting from AI enhancements. Optimal distribution of medical supplies, personnel, and emergency services can make a huge difference, especially in underserved or remote communities. AI systems analyze supply chain data alongside health demand forecasts to ensure resources are where they are needed most. This improves efficiency, reduces waste, and ensures that critical services reach those who need them most urgently.

Furthermore, AI has the potential to enhance the reach and efficacy of health education at the community level. Digital platforms equipped with AI can deliver personalized health education materials, providing individuals with the information they need to make informed health decisions. AI can also power chatbots and virtual assistants that provide round-the-clock health advice and answer questions about symptoms, preventive measures, or nearby health services. As these technologies become more sophisticated and user-friendly, they will play an integral role in health literacy advancement.

Additionally, AI offers opportunities for fostering community connections and support networks. AI-driven platforms can connect individuals with similar health concerns, creating communities of support that facilitate sharing of experiences and solutions. Whether it's a virtual forum for people managing diabetes or an online support group for mental health, AI helps create these spaces where community members can find solidarity and empowerment.

In considering AI for community health, we must also address ethical and privacy concerns, although we delve into these topics in detail in other sections. It's vital to ensure these technologies are deployed equitably and responsibly, so they enhance health outcomes without compromising individual privacy or exacerbating social inequalities. Transparency in AI applications can build trust among community members, encouraging broader adoption and engagement with these innovative solutions.

In conclusion, AI's potential impact on community health is profound and multi-faceted. By predicting outbreaks, personalizing interventions, improving chronic disease management, optimizing resource allocation, enhancing education, and fostering support networks, AI acts as a catalyst for healthier communities. As we eagerly anticipate these changes, it's crucial that we approach the integration of AI into community health with both optimism and caution, ensuring that it is inclusive, ethical, and centered on enhancing the well-being of all individuals. Through thoughtful implementation, AI could very well be the linchpin in achieving widespread and sustainable improvements in public health.

AI-Powered Health Initiatives

Across the globe, artificial intelligence is driving a paradigm shift in community health, extending its transformative influence well beyond the confines of traditional healthcare environments like hospitals and clinics. The burgeoning field of AI-powered health initiatives is focused on enhancing community outreach, prevention strategies, and health education, aiming to create healthier societies through technological innovation.

Central to these initiatives is the utilization of AI to analyze vast datasets, allowing public health officials to identify and predict potential health crises before they manifest on a large scale. For instance, AI algorithms are being deployed to scrutinize patterns of health-related Google searches or social media mentions for early signs of disease outbreaks. This proactive approach can be a game changer, offering the possibility to curtail epidemics by intervening at the earliest possible stage.

In addition, AI is making preventive health measures more accessible and personalized. Take, for example, AI-driven mobile applications designed to educate communities about healthy lifestyle choices. These apps not only disseminate information but also tailor guidance based on individual user data, helping foster behavioral changes that contribute to long-term health improvement. The evolving sophistication of AI also means it can better engage users through interactive and gamified content, turning health education into an engaging, often rewarding experience.

Further still, AI can bridge the gap in healthcare access by providing remote diagnostics and virtual consultation services, ensuring that even people in remote areas have access to expert health advice. These services rely on advanced AI models capable of analyzing input from users, such as symptoms and health history, to suggest possible conditions and next steps. By empowering individuals with AI-assisted tools, communities are better equipped to manage their health autonomously.

In urban settings, AI is being woven into the fabric of city planning to foster healthier living environments. Smart city initiatives leverage AI to optimize everything from traffic management to pollution control. By analyzing data on air quality and population density, AI systems can propose changes in traffic patterns or suggest locations for green spaces, contributing to reduced urban health risks.

AI-powered health initiatives also extend to food supply and nutrition. Advances in AI have enabled the development of systems that can monitor and optimize agricultural practices, ensuring more nutritious and sustainable food production. These systems help manage resources more efficiently, predict crop yields, and mitigate food insecurity, thereby supporting the health of populations at a foundational level.

Beyond individual health benefits, AI is inspiring collective community action through platforms that promote health-focused social enterprises and initiatives. By analyzing social network data, AI can identify key influencers within communities who can champion health-initiated causes, driving awareness and rallying support within their circles. This community-driven approach amplifies the impact of health initiatives, making them more likely to succeed.

Educational institutions are also stepping into the realm of AI-powered health initiatives, integrating AI in their health sciences curricula to prepare future leaders for the challenges of a health landscape increasingly intertwined with technology. Students learn how to harness AI technologies to address community health issues, instilling an understanding of the ethical considerations and potential biases inherent in these systems.

These initiatives are not without their challenges. There are important discussions underway about the ethics of data use and privacy, as well as the pivotal role of equitable AI development to prevent biases against marginalized groups. It's vital that these concerns are addressed to ensure that AI technologies contribute positively and fairly to all areas of public health.

The potential for AI to create healthier communities is immense, yet it calls for a collaborative effort from technologists, healthcare professionals, policymakers, and the communities themselves. By fostering partnerships across sectors, AI-powered health initiatives can be tailored to meet the unique needs of diverse populations, driving forward a future where everyone has the opportunity to lead a healthier life.

Ultimately, the promise of AI-powered health initiatives lies in their ability to inspire a new era of proactive, inclusive, and equitable healthcare beyond traditional settings. They hold the potential not only to transform individual health outcomes but also to redefine collective well-being in a way that is informed by real-time data and supported by universal accessibility. As AI continues to evolve, its role in health initiatives will surely expand, offering new tools for building resilient, health-centric communities worldwide.

Conclusion

The journey through the realms of artificial intelligence (AI) in healthcare reveals a transformative landscape that stretches far beyond what many could have imagined just a few decades ago. AI is not merely an add-on to existing technological frameworks; it is the catalyst reshaping the very foundation of medical practices worldwide. From revolutionizing diagnostics and treatments to reshaping surgeries and patient care, the profound impact of AI is evident across all facets of healthcare. The evidence of AI's contributions is not just in its ability to analyze vast amounts of data with precision but in its potential to personalize care for each individual. This has created a paradigm shift, emphasizing the value of personalized medicine and individualized patient journeys.

We've witnessed AI's prowess in diagnostics, where its accuracy in interpreting medical imagery is unmatched. The innovations in AI tools have enabled medical professionals to detect diseases such as cancer at early stages, where treatment success rates are significantly higher. This accuracy enhances not only patient outcomes but also instills greater confidence in healthcare systems. Meanwhile, AI-driven treatments have brought forth personalized medicine, a realm where treatment plans are tailored to the individual's unique genetic makeup and lifestyle. This is no longer the distant future; it's today's reality, one that offers a life-changing promise to patients around the globe.

In the operating room, AI has significantly enhanced surgical precision. Robots armed with AI capabilities allow surgeons to perform highly intricate operations with unparalleled accuracy, reducing recovery times and increasing patient safety. The integration of AI in surgery is a testament to the technology's ability to redefine what was once deemed impossible, opening doors to new surgical techniques and procedures.

Moreover, the coupling of AI with radiology has sparked a new era for imaging techniques. AI's role in interpreting images extends beyond human capability, identifying subtle changes and abnormalities that might evade even the most experienced radiologists. This collaboration between AI and healthcare professionals not only elevates the quality of diagnostic care but also streamlines workflows, allowing practitioners to focus more on patient interaction and less on administrative tasks.

AI's influence doesn't stop at the diagnostics lab or the surgical suite. It's making strides in drug discovery, where it accelerates the development of new pharmaceuticals, cutting down the time from concept to market. By analyzing biological data with immense precision, AI is fostering innovations in pharmacology that have the potential to eradicate diseases that once posed insurmountable challenges.

Patient care, especially for chronic conditions, has also benefited immensely from AI advancements. Through continuous monitoring and data analysis, AI empowers patients and physicians alike, enabling proactive disease management and intervention. For instance, in diabetes and cardiovascular health, AI-driven tools offer real-time tracking and insights that adjust treatment plans dynamically, improving patient adherence and outcomes.

Furthermore, the intricate dance between AI and mental health is paving the way for more empathetic care. The technology bridges gaps in traditional treatment by offering analytical insights into mental disorders, while innovations continue to push AI towards understanding emotional nuances, striving to complement human empathy.

The ethical considerations surrounding AI in healthcare cannot be understated. As we embrace these technological advancements, it's crucial to navigate the complexities of privacy, data security, and bias in AI algorithms. Ethical AI deployment ensures that the benefits are equitable and that patient trust remains unwavering.

As telemedicine continues to flourish, AI becomes an essential player, expanding access to care and bringing health services to the most remote corners of the world. Here, AI-driven platforms redefine patient-provider interactions with innovations in virtual health, ensuring that geographical barriers no longer impede access to quality care.

AI also streamlines healthcare administration, mitigating burdens on healthcare providers and allowing them to focus more on patient care rather than paperwork. This enhancement in operational efficiency reflects AI's potential to revitalize healthcare infrastructure globally.

The role of AI extends to emergency medicine, where rapid response capabilities save lives during critical scenarios, and in rehabilitation, where adaptive technologies enhance recovery pathways for various conditions. In fighting infectious diseases, AI plays a pivotal role in tracking and contributing effectively to pandemic responses, demonstrating its importance in public health initiatives.

In education and training, AI equips the next generation of healthcare professionals with interactive, immersive learning experiences, preparing them for an AI-driven world. Global health projects further leverage AI to bridge gaps in access and deliver tailored healthcare solutions across diverse populations.

Looking forward, the fusion of AI and precision medicine promises an exciting frontier. As visionary projects unfold and AI becomes entrenched in everyday practice, we expect a future where healthcare is not only more efficient but also more personalized and human-centric. Innovations in elderly and pediatric care highlight AI's capacity to adapt to the needs of different age groups, enhancing quality of life across the spectrum of demographics.

Public perception plays a crucial role in this transformative journey. Understanding societal views and fostering acceptance are paramount in ensuring AI's potential is fully harnessed. Circumventing fears and cultivating trust will be the bedrock upon which AI in healthcare continues to flourish.

This comprehensive journey underscores AI as a monumental force in reshaping global healthcare, whether inside hospital walls or beyond them. Yet, challenges remain, and overcoming technological barriers and regulatory landscapes is paramount to realizing AI's full potential. The promise of AI doesn't merely lie in innovation; it's rooted in the vision of a better, more inclusive healthcare future—an endeavor that continuously beckons our collective commitment.

Appendix A: Appendix

This appendix serves as an essential resource, providing additional insights and a deeper understanding of the transformative role that artificial intelligence is playing in the evolution of healthcare. In this section, we will synthesize information, offer clarifications, and address frequently asked questions that may arise from the preceding chapters. As the embrace of AI in medicine continues to expand, it becomes increasingly important to have a repository of knowledge that reflects the dynamic and constantly evolving nature of this field.

The potential of AI in healthcare is both vast and varied, touching on numerous aspects of medical science and patient care. From revolutionizing diagnostics to personalizing treatment plans, AI holds promises that are gradually unfolding into concrete realities. The appendix aims to supplement the book's main content by ensuring that critical themes and concepts are accessible to a broad audience, from medical professionals to the tech-savvy patient.

Defining Key Terms

Throughout this book, we've encountered various technical terms and concepts integral to understanding AI's impact on healthcare. Here, we clarify some of those terms:

Machine Learning: A subset of AI that enables computers to learn from data without being explicitly programmed. In healthcare, it helps to predict patient outcomes based on historical data.

Neural Networks: Modeled after the human brain, these systems are designed to recognize patterns and interpret sensory data.

Big Data: Large volumes of data that, when analyzed with AI tools, can reveal trends and patterns, particularly useful in making informed healthcare decisions.

Precision Medicine: An innovative approach that considers individual variability in genes, environment, and lifestyle for each person.

Expanding Further

When delving into AI's role in healthcare, a crucial element is understanding not only the technological capabilities but also the ethical and practical considerations involved. The appendix serves as a bridge, connecting the technical advancements covered in the book with their real-world implications, fostering a broader appreciation of the challenges and opportunities that lie ahead.

AI's advancements prompt questions about data privacy, algorithmic bias, and the evolving role of healthcare professionals. These topics merit ongoing discussion and reflective thought, underscoring the importance of an informed and engaged readership ready to grapple with the complexities introduced by AI in medicine.

By distilling the book's core concepts and supplementing them with this additional context, the appendix aims to inspire readers to critically engage with the material and contribute to the broader dialogue surrounding AI and its place in the future of healthcare.